Quick Cognitive Screening for Clinicians

Mini Mental, Clock Drawing and Other Brief Tests

Quick Cognitive Screening for Clinicians

Mini Mental, Clock Drawing and Other Brief Tests

Kenneth I Shulman MD SM FRCPsych FRCPC

Professor and Richard Lewar Chair
Department of Psychiatry
University of Toronto
Sunnybrook and Women's College Health Sciences Centre
Toronto, Ontario, Canada

Anthony Feinstein MPhil PhD FRCPC

Professor
Department of Psychiatry
University of Toronto
Sunnybrook and Women's College Health Sciences Centre
Toronto, Ontario, Canada

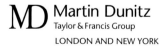
Martin Dunitz
Taylor & Francis Group
LONDON AND NEW YORK

© 2003 Martin Dunitz, an imprint of the Taylor & Francis Group

First published in the United Kingdom in 2003
by Martin Dunitz, an imprint of the Taylor and Francis Group, 11 New Fetter
Lane, London EC4P 4EE

Tel.: +44 (0) 20 7583 9855
Fax.: +44 (0) 20 7842 2298
E-mail: info@dunitz.co.uk
Website: http://www.dunitz.co.uk

**WM
145.5
.N4
S562q
2003**

Although every effort has been made to ensure that all owners of copyright material have been acknowledged in this publication, we would be glad to acknowledge in subsequent reprints or editions any omissions brought to our attention.

Although every effort has been made to ensure that drug doses and other information are presented accurately in this publication, the ultimate responsibility rests
with the prescribing physician. Neither the publishers nor the authors can be
held responsible for errors or for any consequences arising from the use of
information contained herein. For detailed prescribing information or instructions on the use of any product or procedure discussed herein, please consult the
prescribing information or instructional material issued by the manufacturer.

A CIP record for this book is available from the British Library.

ISBN 1 84184 239 7

Distributed in the USA by
Fulfilment Center
Taylor & Francis
10650 Tobben Drive
Independence, KY 41051, USA
Toll Free Tel.: +1 800 634 7064
E-mail: taylorandfrancis@thomsonlearning.com

Distributed in Canada by
Taylor & Francis
74 Rolark Drive
Scarborough, Ontario M1R 4G2, Canada
Toll Free Tel.: +1 877 226 2237
E-mail: tal_fran@istar.ca

Distributed in the rest of the world by
Thomson Publishing Services
Cheriton House
North Way
Andover, Hampshire SP10 5BE, UK
Tel.: +44 (0)1264 332424
E-mail: salesorder.tandf@thomsonpublishingservices.co.uk

Composition by EXPO Holdings, Malaysia

Printed and bound in Great Britain by The Cromwell Press Ltd

Cover image reproduced from Shulman (2000) *Int J Ger Psychiatry* **15**: 548–561
with permission from John Wiley & Sons Ltd.

Contents

Preface

This collaboration on cognitive screening brings together two rapidly growing and overlapping fields, namely geriatric psychiatry and neuropsychiatry. As colleagues in the same department, we came to realize the importance of sharing our expertise and experience of assessing and treating a wide range of central nervous system (CNS) disorders. The fields of psychiatry, geriatrics, neurology, neuropsychology and primary care all share a role and vested interest in the early identification of brain disorders as well as having the capacity to monitor cognitive changes over time.

The book focuses on the brief or 'quick' cognitive screening instruments. Inevitably, there is a selection bias on the part of the authors in terms of which instruments we chose to review and their relative emphasis. However, we did strive for objectivity in reviewing those instruments most widely used and studied. We also felt that a chapter devoted to frontal lobe tests was necessary, given the importance of this brain region in modulating behavior and cognition. In this book, we summarize the current state of knowledge related to the development of cognitive screening instruments. Hopefully, readers will find the book of academic interest and practical value in their daily clinical work.

Kenneth I Shulman
Anthony Feinstein

Acknowledgements

We gratefully acknowledge the help of Dilshad Ratansi in the preparation of the manuscript and Abigail Griffin for her careful editing of the text.

Dedication

We dedicate this book to our families:
Karen, Pippa, Saul and Clara
Rhona, Rayzie and Tamara

chapter 1

Introduction to cognitive screening

Why cognitive screening?

With a rapidly growing elderly population comes the 'demographic imperative' that neuropsychiatric disorders will become one of the major clinical and public health challenges of the next generation. The dementias and neuropsychiatric disorders in this population, as well as in younger patients, represents a challenge for which we are still largely unprepared. While many of these conditions are not reversible, secondary and tertiary prevention are realistic and important goals for health-care systems around the world. Prevention involves early diagnosis and treatment, but also disability limitation and the prevention of complications resulting from those disorders (Ganguli, 1997). Ganguli rightly makes the point that 'No cognitive screening measure is an Alzheimer's test'. While non-professionals can generally perform screening, those who test positive need to be targeted for more skilled and detailed assessments. Although screening represents only the first step in a process of assessment and 'work-up', it still offers the best opportunity for secondary prevention (Ganguli, 1997).

Early detection carries with it a number of important potential benefits from a clinical as well as a societal perspective:

1. The early diagnosis of a neuropsychiatric or dementing disorder offers the opportunity to provide an explanation to patients and

families regarding changes in cognition, functioning, behavior or mood.

2. The establishment of a firm diagnosis allows for planning of important issues for the patient and family. This includes the preparation of Powers of Attorney for property and personal care; Living Wills for end-of-life care; Last Will and Testament for the distribution of one's assets according to personal wishes; as well as planning for an appropriate residential facility which may become necessary for care in the future.

3. The establishment of a diagnosis of dementia or other brain disorder identifies an increased risk for delirium and also highlights the need to monitor the risks for driving and taking appropriate action.

4. There have been significant advances in the treatment of cognitive impairment with cognitive enhancers such as cholinesterase inhibitors (Herrmann, 2002). The earlier the diagnosis is established, the more likely it is that these drugs may provide benefit by retarding the progression of the disease, in some cases temporarily improving function.

5. The costs of these disorders from a societal perspective are substantial and threaten to overwhelm the health-care system in the next generation. The appropriate planning of services will help to minimize societal costs, although this will not prevent the inevitable increase in costs associated with this growing population (Ostbye and Cross, 1994). This planning includes paying close attention to the needs of caregivers.

6. Secondary opportunities from a societal perspective include the development of standards for dementia care and the development of strategies for population-based health care of cognitively impaired individuals and their caregivers (Lorentz et al, 2002).

7. Finally, from an academic perspective, early detection and diagnosis of dementia will allow for the participation of individuals in clinical research at a relatively early stage and thereby allow important testing of a variety of innovative therapeutic interventions.

Screening may also be helpful in identifying those individuals suffering from 'mild cognitive impairment' (Geda and Petersen, 2001). These are individuals who typically have memory complaints, corroborated by an informant, but whose cognitive impairment is not sufficiently severe to establish a diagnosis of dementia. Cognitive screening may identify such individuals for long-term follow-up or possible pharmacological intervention. As clinical trials are underway in this population, it may be increasingly important to determine which factors associated with mild cognitive impairment predict who will go on to develop a progressive dementia.

Another important function of brief cognitive tests is not simply initial screening but also monitoring of change in cognition over time. Since diagnosis is often unclear after initial assessment, the capacity to retest over the course of follow-up is clinically very useful.

Freyne (2001) cautions that there are potential drawbacks to screening and that it is not an entirely benign procedure. False-positive results may cause distress and lead to the stigma of being labeled mentally ill. Furthermore, in many jurisdictions a lack of specialized neuropsychiatric, geriatric and psychogeriatric services may raise serious questions about the capacity to manage positive cases identified through a screening mechanism.

Who to screen?

In general, screening should be carried out in a population of individuals who yield the highest potential of identifying the disorder (Ganguli, 1997). This inevitably means those who have achieved great age, where the prevalence of dementia is highest, especially those 80 and over (CSHA, 2000). Others have argued that individuals who have subjective complaints of memory impairment should be screened, but there are two problems with this approach. The first is the difficulty of anosognosia, which prevents individuals who suffer from dementia from identifying their own deficits (Sevush and Leve, 1993). The second is that those who complain of subjective impairment of memory also have a high prevalence of depression (Tobianski et al, 1995). This notion is countered by the recent work of Alexopoulos et al (1993), who found that reversible dementia or 'pseudodementia' associated with major depression often leads to a dementing illness over time. Increasingly, depression is being recognized as a risk factor for dementia and the original dismissal of subjective impairment of memory concerns may have been premature (Butters et al, 2000; Devenand et al, 1996).

Finally, the group identified by informants as having concerns related to cognition represents an important population for screening. O'Connor et al (1989) showed a direct correlation between dementia severity measured by detailed neuropsychological testing and the ratings by key informants. Indeed, a number of authors suggest that informant questionnaires can be successfully incorporated into formal cognitive screening (Jorm, 1997). Furthermore, there is some evidence to suggest that the combination of cognitive testing with informant reports increases the accuracy of detecting true cases of dementia (MacKinnon and Mulligan, 1998) (see Chapter 8 on Informant questionnaires).

Obstacles to screening

Considerable evidence suggests that there are high rates of missed dementia diagnoses in primary care settings (Borson et al, 2000). Moreover, a recent study found that dementia was missed in 67% of all affected cases and in over 90% when impairment was only mild in severity (Valcour et al, 2000). So why is cognitive screening not implemented as widely as one would expect?

Bush et al (1997) have reviewed the major obstacles to cognitive screening in general practice. While general practitioners acknowledge and recognize the importance of cognitive screening, they cite lack of time as one of the principal obstacles to screening in a general practice setting. Given that the length of a primary care visit varies from 7.5 to 19 minutes (Lorentz et al, 2002), it is unlikely that a screen that requires more than 3 or 4 minutes would be utilized. For example, the widely known Mini-Mental State Examination (MMSE), which takes about 10 minutes on average to administer, is unlikely to be utilized on a routine basis. If screening is to be utilized in such a setting, then screening tests need to be less than 5 minutes in duration in order to find practical application at the front lines of the health service (Lorentz et al, 2002).

The other concern expressed by general practitioners is that of acceptability. Many cognitive screening tests risk offending patients and this would deter general practitioners and other primary care clinicians from routinely testing cognition. Nonetheless, the general practitioners in the study by Bush et al (1997) indicated that, if a screening test proved to be 'effective', acceptable and brief, the vast majority would attempt to use it on a routine basis. If the intent is to increase the identification of individuals vulnerable to a dementia or other neuropsychiatric disorder, then identification by frontline clinicians is critical.

Qualities of an ideal screening test

Lorentz et al (2000) note that screening instruments tend to perform best when the target sample is heavily weighted with individuals suffering from severe cognitive impairment. Therefore, tests evaluated in different samples will not be directly comparable. Ideally, tests should be validated against a diagnostic standard that is applied both to subjects with and to subjects without dementia and includes those with mild levels of impairment. Effort should also be made to validate screening instruments in sample populations that include a broad range of educational levels and a wide mix of ethnic and cultural backgrounds. It has been recommended that cognitive screening tests should be formally compared in order to choose between them. Receiver operating characteristic (ROC) curves are the best methodology for doing this (Storey et al, 2001; Stuss et al, 1996).

Factors other than cognitive impairment can influence test scores (Ganguli, 1997). These factors need to be taken into account when screening is carried out in the absence of any other knowledge of the individual. Factors such as education, cultural and linguistic differences, as well as sensory impairment, can significantly affect test scores. Nonetheless, clinicians need to be aware of potential confounders before pursuing detailed assessment and investigation in individuals who screen positive. Cognitive screening instruments should be influenced as little as possible by these variables.

The ideal screening test should be:

- very brief (less than 2 to 3 minutes in a primary care setting)
- well tolerated and acceptable to patients without producing excessive defensiveness or catastrophic reactions
- easy to administer and score
- relatively independent of confounding factors such as education, culture and language
- possessing excellent psychometric properties including inter-rater and test/retest reliability, good sensitivity and specificity and high positive and negative predictive validity
- able to cover a wide range of intellectual functions, i.e. cast a wide net

Ultimately, there is no 'perfect' cognitive screening test or battery. The search for the test or battery with the best psychometric properties must be balanced against the practical issue of implementation. If primary care physicians and other busy clinicians will not implement a test because it is too long, too cumbersome or unacceptable, then it is not an effective screening test. It may be necessary to compromise on the psychometric properties for the sake of having a test that will be utilized in order to identify those who are in need of further assessment. As long as there is no misconception that the screening test is 'diagnostic' or permanently labels anyone as 'demented' or cognitively impaired, then one can safely and comfortably implement a compromise approach to screening.

Consideration must be given to practical issues in reviewing the role of cognitive screening (Freyne, 2001). Specifically, the resource implications at both primary and secondary levels need to be addressed as well as the careful selection of appropriate and effective screening instruments. Certainly, there is little support for screening of all elderly people in a general population (Brodaty et al, 1998). However, Freyne (2001) acknowledges that 'opportunistic case finding and screening of specific groups can be useful'. She calls for further pilot studies that address

Table 1.1 Guidelines for development of screening programs (from Freyne, 2001, with permission from the Royal Society of Medicine).

1. The condition being sought is serious
2. There should be acceptable treatment for people with the condition
3. Facilities for diagnosis and treatment should be available
4. There should be a recognized latent (or early symptomatic) stage
5. The natural history of the disease should be understood
6. There should be a sensitive and specific test
7. The test should be acceptable to the population
8. There should be an agreed policy on who to treat as patients
9. Cost of case finding should be economically balanced in relation to overall expenditure in the screening process

Case finding should be a continuous process, not an isolated incident.

screening questions and strengthen links between primary and secondary care services. This is an initial step in identifying the barriers to screening and the practical obstacles that need to be overcome for screening to be implemented. It would be well to keep in mind guidelines for the development of screening programs as originally described by Wilson and Junger (1968) (Table 1.1).

Definitions of psychometric properties

These definitions are from Hennekens and Buring (1987). The validity of a screening test is measured by its ability to do what it is supposed to do, that is, correctly categorize persons who have preclinical disease as test-positive and those without preclinical disease as test-negative. Table 1.2 summarizes the relationship between the results of a screening test and the actual presence of disease as determined by the results of an appropriate subsequent diagnostic test.

Sensitivity and specificity are two measures of the validity of a screening test. Sensitivity is defined as the probability of testing positive if the

Table 1.2 Results of a screening test (from Hennekens and Buring, 1987, with permission from Lippincott Williams and Wilkins).

	Disease status (Dx) ('truth')		
	Positive	*Negative*	*Total*
Results of screening test (T)			
Positive	a	b	a + b
Negative	c	d	c + d
Total	a + c	b + d	

Sensitivity = Probability $(T^+|Dx^+)$ = $\dfrac{a}{a+c}$

Specificity = Probability $(T^-|Dx^-)$ = $\dfrac{d}{b+d}$

PV^+ = Probability $(Dx^+|T^+)$ = $\dfrac{a}{a+b}$

PV^- = Probability $(Dx^-|T^-)$ = $\dfrac{d}{c+d}$

a = The number of individuals for whom the screening test is positive and the individual actually has the disease (true positive).

b = The number for whom the screening test is positive but the individual does not have the disease (false positive).

c = The number for whom the screening test is negative but the individual does have the disease (false negative).

d = The number for whom the screening test is negative and the individual does not have the disease (true negative).

disease is truly present and is calculated by a/(a + c) (Table 1.2). As the sensitivity of a test increases, the number of persons with the disease who are missed by being incorrectly classified as test-negative (false negatives) will decrease. Specificity is defined as the probability of screening negative if the disease is truly absent and is calculated by d/(b + d). A highly specific test will rarely be positive in the absence of disease and will therefore result in a lower proportion of persons without disease who are incorrectly classified as test-positive (false positives).

ROC curves are useful in describing the accuracy of a screening test over a range of cut-off points (Jarvenpaa et al, 2002). Moreover, the ROC curve can serve as a nomogram for determining specificity corresponding with a given sensitivity. It demonstrates the clear trade off between sensitivity and specificity for cognitive screening tests and therefore can be helpful in determining the best cut-off point. The area under the ROC curve best describes the accuracy of the test. The larger the area under the curve, the better the psychometric properties of this test. Throughout the book we will report and provide ROC curves to reflect the accuracy and validity of various tests and instruments.

With respect to the yield (Hennekens and Buring, 1987), or number of cases detected by a screening program, one measure that is commonly considered is the predictive value of the screening test (Vecchio, 1966). Predictive value measures whether or not an individual actually has the disease, given the results of the screening test. Predictive value positive (PV$^+$) is the probability that a person actually has the disease given that he or she tests positive, and is calculated (using the notation in Table 1.2) as:

$$PV^+ = \frac{a}{a+b}$$

The positive predictive value is dependent on the prevalence of the disorder in the population being studied. Analogously, predictive value negative (PV$^-$) is the probability that an individual is truly disease-free given a negative screening test, and is calculated as follows:

$$PV^- = \frac{d}{c+d}$$

References

Alexopoulos GS, Meyer BS, Young RC, Mattis S, Kakuma T (1993) The course of geriatric depression with reversible dementia: a controlled study. *Am J Psychiatry* **150**:1693–1699.

Borson S, Scanlan JM, Brush M, Vitaliano PP, Dokmak A (2000) The Mini-Cog: A cognitive 'vital signs' measure for dementia screening in multi-lingual elderly. *Int J Geriatr Psychiatry* **15**:1021–1027.

Brodaty H, Clarke J, Ganguli M, et al (1998) Screening for cognitive impairment in general practice: Toward a consensus. *Alzheimer Dis Assoc Disord* 12:1–13.

Bush C, Kozak J, Elmslie T (1997) Screening for cognitive impairment in the elderly. *Can Fam Physician* 43:1763–1768.

Butters MA, Becker JT, Nebes RD, Zmuda MD, Mulsant BH, et al (2000) Changes in cognitive functioning following treatment of late-life depression. *Am J Psychiatry* 157:1949–1954.

Canadian Study of Health and Aging Working Group (2000) The incidence of dementia in Canada. *Neurology* 55:66–73.

Devanand DP, Sano M, Tang M-X, Taylor S, Gurland BG, et al (1996) Depressed mood and the incidence of Alzheimer's disease in the elderly living in the community. *Arch Gen Psychiatry* 53:175–182.

Freyne A (2001) Screening for dementia in primary care – a viable proposition? *Irish J Psych Med* 18(2):75–77.

Ganguli M (1997) The use of screening instruments for the detection of dementia. *Neuroepidemiology* 16:271–280.

Geda YE, Petersen RC (2001) Clinical trials in mild cognitive impairment. In Gauthier S, Cummings JL (eds) *Alzheimer's Disease and Related Disorders Annual*. London: Martin Dunitz, 69–83.

Hennekens CH, Buring JE (1987) Screening. In Maurent SL (ed) *Epidemiology in Medicine*. Boston: Little Brown, 327–347.

Herrmann N (2002) Cognitive phamacotherapy of Alzheimer's disease and other dementias. *Can J Psychiatry* 47(8):715–722.

Jarvenpaa T, Rinne JO, Raiha I, Koskenvuo MK, Lopponen M, et al (2002) Characteristics of two telephone screens for cognitive impairment. *Dement Geriatr Cogn Disord* 13:149–155.

Jorm AF (1997) Methods of screening for dementia: A meta-analysis of studies comparing an informant questionnaire with a brief cognitive test. *Alzheimer's Dis Assoc Disord* 11(3):158–162.

Lorentz WJ, Scanlan JM, Borson S (2002) Brief screening tests for dementia. *Can J Psychiatry* 47(8):723–733.

MacKinnon A, Mulligan R (1998) Combining cognitive testing and informant report to increase accuracy in screening for dementia. *Am J Psychiatry* 155: 1529–1535.

O'Connor DW, Pollitt PA, Treasure FP, et al (1989) The influence of education, social class and sex on Mini-Mental State scores. *Psychol Med* 19:771–776.

Ostbye T, Cross E (1994) Net economic costs of dementia in Canada. *Can Med Assoc J* 151:1457–1464.

Sevush S, Leve N (1993) Denial of memory deficits in Alzheimer's Disease. *Am J Psychiatry* 150:748–751.

Storey JE, Rowland JT, Basic D, Conforti DA (2001) A comparison of five clock scoring methods using ROC (receiver operating characteristic) curve analysis. *Int J Geriatr Psychiatry* 16:394–399.

Stuss DT, Meiran N, Guzman A, Lafleche G, Wilmer J (1996) Do long tests yield a more accurate diagnosis of dementia than short tests? A comparison of 5 neuropsychological tests. *Arch Neurol* 1996;53:1033–1039.

Tobianski R, Blizard R, Livingston G, Mann A (1995) The Gospel Oak Study Stage IV: The clinical relevance of subjective memory impairment in older people. *Psychol Med* 25:779–786.

Valcour VG, Masaki KH, Curb JD, Blanchette PL (2000) The detection of dementia in the primary care setting. *Arch Intern Med* **160**:2964–2968.

Vecchio TJ (1966) Predictive value of a single diagnostic test in unselected populations. *N Engl J Med* **271**:1171–1173.

Wilson J, Junger G (1968) The principles and practice of screening for disease. *Public Health Papers* **34**:26–39.

chapter 2

Premorbid intellectual functioning

Intelligence

As an introduction to a chapter describing the assessment of premorbid intelligence, a few comments on the question of intelligence *per se* are needed. Intelligence comprises many different abilities and, as such, the majority of approaches to assessment comprise sets of different tasks, both verbal and performance related. The most widely used measures are the Wechsler Intelligence Scales (Wechsler, 1981) which have gone through periodic revisions since their introduction. Single-scale measures of intelligence such as the Raven's Progressive Matrices (Raven, 1996) are used less frequently, although in certain circumstances they may be preferred.

Intelligence tests are scored and provide a scaled index of intelligence, with 100 taken as the mean and 15 as the standard deviation. Approximately 95% of the population will have an intelligence score within two standard deviations of the mean, establishing the 'normal' intelligence quotient (IQ) range as 70–130.

This intellectual index is not, however, all-embracing of human attributes (Spreen and Strauss,1998). Wisdom, practical knowledge and social skills, to mention but three, are not captured by these tests. Similarly, while IQ is an important predictor of school grades, it accounts for no more than a quarter of the overall variance when it comes to predicting academic success, with other factors such as persistence, application and motivation proving equally, or more, important.

Premorbid IQ

Before beginning a cognitive examination it is important to have an estimate of premorbid intellectual ability as a yardstick with which to
measure possible decline. To provide such an estimate requires a test
that is relatively robust to cognitive impairment and able to withstand
the destructive effects of degenerative diseases such as senile dementia of
the Alzheimer type or Lewy body dementia. In subjects with acquired
brain disease, performance aspects of IQ may be more adversely affected
than verbal abilities, thereby providing a clue as to the greater potential
resilience of verbal aspects of cognition. Even within the verbal domain,
certain aspects of cognition are more robust than others. Thus, verbal
comprehension and aspects of verbal expression decline moderately in
patients with dementing illnesses. Similarly, reading comprehension
may also decline. On the other hand, reading ability for irregular words
is better preserved (Cummings et al, 1986). This observation led Nelson
and O'Connell (1978) to develop the National Adult Reading Test
(NART).

The National Adult Reading Test

The NART is made up of 50 orthographically irregular words. The
subject is required to read them aloud in an order of decreasing frequency of usage. The emphasis is on pronunciation, which depends on
familiarity from previous exposure. The number of errors made (words
mispronounced) are tallied and used to generate an IQ score. The NART
was originally standardized against the Wechsler Adult Intelligence Scale
(WAIS) (Nelson, 1982) and more recently against the WAIS-Revised
(WAIS-R) on a sample of subjects aged 18–70 years (Nelson and Willison,
1991). On the basis of NART scores, the examiner can predict both a
WAIS-R full-scale IQ ranging from 69 to 131 and a WAIS-R verbal IQ
ranging from 70 to 127.

What makes a reading test such a useful marker of premorbid intellect
is that NART scores do not correlate with age or socioeconomic status.

While cognition declines with age, with impairments in memory and attention beginning as early as the fifth decade (Feinstein et al, 1994), the NART is fairly resistant to the effects of aging up until 84 years (Brayne and Beardsall, 1990). Furthermore, the NART may still provide a valid indicator of premorbid IQ, even in patients in the early stages (Crawford et al, 1988; Cummings et al, 1986; Nebes et al, 1984; O'Carroll and Gilleard, 1986) and later stages (Hart et al, 1986; Nelson and McKenna, 1975; Nelson and O'Connell, 1978) of Alzheimer's disease.

There are, however, a number of reports suggesting that the NART may not be accurate in patients with dementia, even in those at the milder end of the spectrum. O'Carroll et al (1995) challenged the assumption that reading ability at the level of a single word is maintained despite increasing dementia. In a study of 68 patients with probable Alzheimer dementia of varying severity, significant, albeit moderate, correlations were noted between NART scores and those on the Mini-Mental State Examination (MMSE) (Folstein et al, 1975). When the authors divided the sample according to dementia severity, with subgroups matched for age, sex and years of education, significant differences in NART scores between groups were revealed. The study concluded that NART scores were predicated by dementia severity and provided a serious underestimation of premorbid IQ in subjects with a MMSE score of less than 13.

Further evidence along these lines comes from Patterson et al (1994) who also noted a close correlation between severity of dementia and NART scores, with the added caveat that the NART may fall short by up to 15 points in estimating premorbid IQ in individuals with moderately severe dementia.

Longitudinal validity studies of the NART demonstrate mixed results. In a sample of 61 healthy normal adults tested twice, 10 days apart, there was a significant but small decrease in errors at the second testing, which prompted the conclusion that practice effects were minimal and most likely clinically unimportant (Crawford et al, 1989a). However, in a second study with a 1-year test–retest interval and comprising a sample of 69 community-resident, non-dementing adults, a significant decrease in errors was found, highlighting the role of practice effects (J. Cockburn, Doctoral Thesis). The results from studies involving demented patients are equally equivocal. In a 1-year longitudinal study of subjects with mild to moderate dementia, a fall-off in cognitive performance was not matched by a similar decrease in NART scores, suggesting a dissociation between reading ability and other aspects of cognition as dementia progresses (O'Carroll et al, 1987). The authors cautioned that this result may not hold for more severe forms of dementia. Two further studies revealed that this was indeed the case. A 3-year study of patients with probable Alzheimer's disease noted a deterioration in NART scores over time with a discernible pattern in deficits, i.e. regularization in word pronunciation (e.g. capon becoming 'cap on'), suggesting a loss of semantic memory in the presence of intact phonological ability (Fromm et al, 1991). Another longitudinal study (Paque and Warrington, 1995) of 57 Alzheimer patients produced results that straddled both of these earlier studies. With a 10-month test–retest interval, an average 5-point decline in NART scores was notably less than a 10-point decline in verbal IQ and 8-point decline in performance IQ, suggesting a relative resilience rather than a preservation in reading abilities. Methodological weaknesses in these studies have been noted and include the use of a shortened version of the NART and the fact that subjects were tested on no more than two occasions. In order to address these concerns, a detailed assessment of the NART's resilience to decay over a 4-year period was undertaken in a sample of 78 patients whose diagnosis of dementia was either confirmed at autopsy (n = 50) or made clinically (n = 28). In addition to annual NART examinations, subjects were seen every 4 months for a behavioral assessment, at which point the MMSE was also completed (Cockburn et al, 2000). A mean MMSE of 14.3 on entry to the study attests to a significant degree of cognitive impairment in the sample. The gist of the serial results is that the MMSE and NART scores declined over time, with the extent of the NART decline a function of the MMSE score on entry into the study, i.e. the more pronounced the dementia, the more rapid the longitudinal decline in NART scores.

The validity of the NART has been examined in other dementing conditions.

Korsakoff's syndrome

There are a number of studies that have used the NART to estimate pre-morbid intelligence in Korsakoff patients (Jacobson et al, 1990; Joyce and Robbins, 1991; Kopelman 1989, 1991; Leng and Parkin, 1988; Mayes et al, 1991; Shoqeirat and Mayes, 1991; Shoqeirat et al, 1990) despite evidence that the disease may affect word pronunciation. Crawford et al, (1988) found that 12 Korsakoff patients (alcohol related) made more NART errors than control subjects matched for age, sex and years of education. A second study subsequently replicated the result in a larger sample of Korsakoff patients once again matched with healthy controls. Of note was that only Korsakoff patients made more NART errors, but that the NART correlated significantly with memory impairment and was less sensitive than demographic variables in predicting premorbid intellect (O'Carroll et al, 1992a). This result is perplexing, given that general intellect in Korsakoff patients is intact in the face of significant memory impairment. One possible explanation relates to the impulsivity of Korsakoff patients which incorporates an inability to error-check coupled with the blurting-out of responses typical of confabulators (O'Carroll et al, 1992a).

Huntington's disease

There are two studies that have used the NART in subjects with Huntington's disease and both have raised doubts about the validity of the test (Blackmore et al, 1994; Crawford et al, 1988). This has raised the question (yet to be answered) of whether demographic variables are not perhaps more sensitive indicators of premorbid intelligence.

Schizophrenia

The NART has been used to assess premorbid ability in patients with schizophrenia (Dunkley and Rogers, 1994; Jones et al, 1994), although there is evidence that in one subgroup of patients results may be problematic. In a study that compared results in community-based and long-stay institutional schizophrenic patients, NART scores in the latter were considered severely compromised despite close between-group demographic matching (Crawford et al, 1992). Two possibilities could explain this result: the long-stay patients may indeed have had a lower premorbid IQ, a factor that may have predisposed them to chronic institutionalization in the first place; or alternatively, the NART performance was affected by the disease, which in the case of hospital-bound patients may have been a more severe variant. Given this finding, the use of the NART in schizophrenic patients is probably safest in those who are acutely ill. Empirical evidence for this comes from a study that failed to detect differences in NART scores between 20 acutely ill, non-medicated schizophrenic patients and 20 control subjects (O'Carroll et al, 1992b).

Depression

There is a weak consensus that depression does not affect the accuracy of irregular word pronunciation (Austin et al, 1992; Crawford et al, 1987). The question of whether the robustness of the NART in the context of depression could then be used to help tease out the diagnostic dilemma of dementia versus pseudodementia (i.e. depression masquerading as dementia) has been summarized by O'Carroll et al (1994). Discrepancies between the NART on the one hand and scores on the WAIS-R, Raven's Matrices and Wechsler Memory Scale on the other have been explored with unsatisfactory results. The NART may therefore be a valid means of testing premorbid IQ in depressed patients, but its use does not extend beyond this.

Traumatic brain injury

There is one study reported in the literature assessing the validity of the NART in subjects with closed-head injury (Watt and O'Carroll, 1999). Comparing three groups of subjects, namely those with a closed traumatic brain injury (TBI) (n = 25), healthy subjects (n = 50) and orthopedic patients (n = 20), no premorbid differences were observed. Of note is the composition of the head-injured sample: 60% had a severe TBI (Glasgow Coma Scale score, 3–8), 24% had a moderately severe TBI (Glasgow Coma Scale score, 9–12) and 16% had a mild injury (Glasgow Coma Scale score, 13–15). Unfortunately, the NART data were not analyzed according to TBI severity, thereby neglecting an important question that has been particularly germane to dementia research in

Alzheimer's disease, namely, does the severity of the pathological process compromise the accuracy of what is being measured?

A further important observation from this TBI study is that, of two other measures of premorbid intellect, i.e. the Cambridge Contextual Reading Test (CCRT) (Beardsall and Huppert, 1994) and the Spot-the-Word Test (SWT) (Baddeley et al, 1993), only the former was considered useful in assessing premorbid intellect in TBI patients.

Glioma

A study of 16 patients with glioma who had received whole-brain prophylactic radiation demonstrated poor performance on the NART relative to a group of demographically matched healthy controls (Ebmeier et al, 1993). The preponderance of tumors in the left temporal lobe in this sample hinders extrapolating this result to all patients who have received similar radical therapy.

Abbreviated NART

The full NART contains 50 words. This has led some investigators to suggest that the length of the test may be anxiety provoking, thereby affecting subjects' performance. A study of a shortened version (Beardsall and Brayne, 1990) demonstrated minimal loss of predictive ability (Crawford et al, 1991). However, there is a consensus amongst researchers that the full version is not a 'threatening' test, given that it taps well-established knowledge. Furthermore, the majority of subjects do not know when they are making an error by mispronouncing a word and, therefore, are unlikely to allow anxiety to intrude into their performance. The abbreviated NART is thus seldom used.

Given the cultural specificity of words used in the NART, a North American version has been developed, the NAART (Blair and Spreen, 1989) or AMNART (Grober and Sliwinski, 1991). A complementary word-reading system is the Wide Range Achievement Test, third edition (WRAT3) (Wilkinson, 1993). Two versions of the WRAT3 are given, thereby mitigating the effects of practice. The reading test consists of two sections, namely a list of 15 letters of the alphabet followed by 42 words. As with the NART, the emphasis is on the correct pronunciation. The words are read first and if subjects score fewer than five correct responses, they must take the letter identification test as well. If, however, there are more than five correct pronunciations, the letter reading can be dispensed with, although credit must be given for this section when calculating the final score. Raw scores are converted into standardized scores that approximate premorbid IQ and grade scores that place the individual at a school grade commensurate with his or her premorbid intellectual ability. The WRAT3 has, in addition to reading sections, others devoted to spelling and arithmetic.

Summarizing the NART data, it is important to note that validity studies have generally targeted healthy subjects or those with probable, possible or definite Alzheimer's disease. To a lesser extent, patients with schizophrenia, TBI, Huntington's disease, depression and one particular type of brain tumor have also been investigated. How similar data stand up in other common dementing conditions such as vascular dementia, Lewy body dementia or the cognitive impairments associated with common disorders such as multiple sclerosis and Parkinson's disease have not been assessed with the same thoroughness. Therefore, any conclusions concerning the NART must be viewed with this limitation in mind. The weight of evidence points to the NART being a valid indicator of premorbid intelligence in healthy individuals and probably those with early onset (and thus less cognitively impaired) Alzheimer's disease. In more severely compromised patients, the evidence suggests that the NART underestimates premorbid intellect, particularly when the MMSE score is less than 13.

Other methods for assessing premorbid IQ

Cambridge Contextual Reading Test

The concerns over the validity of the NART have prompted attempts at developing improved ways of ascertaining premorbid intellect. One approach has been to counteract the possibility that increasing mispronunciation with advancing dementia occurs because individuals fail to recognize words as familiar (Beardsall and Huppert, 1994). Recognition may, however, be fostered by embedding the target word in a sentence that confers context. This semantic association may therefore address not only what Fromm and colleagues (1991) postulated was a deficit in semantic memory that underlay the increasing difficulties demented patients experienced with word pronunciation, but also the potential confounder of poor education. Furthermore, there is evidence that adding a contextual sentence may enhance performance via a different mechanism, namely sentence priming, which is probably intact in demented patients. This refers to meaning derived from the entire sentence rather than from a set of individual word associations.

There is empirical evidence that embedding target words in semantic and syntactic contexts improves NART performance, both in healthy older subjects and in those with minimal and moderate dementia. Of note, is that healthy elderly subjects with average reading skills increased their NART scores by 28% whereas better readers did not benefit from context (Beardsall and Huppert, 1994). The improvements in NART scores for minimally and moderately demented patients were 29 and 39%, respectively.

In a wide-ranging study that attempted to validate the CCRT, Beardsall (1998) enrolled a sample of 73 healthy older subjects (70 years and older) in a protocol that included the CCRT, NART, the verbal subset of the Wechsler Adult Intelligence Scale (vIQ), a detailed set of demographic data and the Mill Hill Vocabulary Test (MHVT) (Raven, 1958), since vocabulary is another putative marker of premorbid IQ (see section on WAIS subscales).

An example of some of the sentences of the CCRT are shown below, with the NART words in italics.

Example 1: The bride was given a beautiful *bouquet* by the *courteous* groom. They began to walk down the *aisle* as the organist played the first *chord* of the *psalm*.

Example 2: The prisoner was *gaoled* for five years, although he said, 'I *deny* all charges against me'.

The results largely replicated the earlier findings, i.e. that the presence of context was most beneficial in boosting the scores of those individuals with the poorest reading ability. These individuals posted a 10%

improvement over their NART scores. The CCRT also showed reasonably strong correlations with the WAIS-R verbal IQ and the Mill Hill Vocabulary Test, thereby illustrating that the test is a valid measure of verbal IQ, at least for British subjects. Furthermore, when the CCRT was entered into a regression analysis with the aim of determining predictors of verbal IQ, it accounted for a respectable 61% of the variance. The author therefore concluded that the CCRT was the preferred method for detecting premorbid intellect in elderly subjects with poor reading skills and those with at least moderately severe dementia.

One further study compared the NART with the CCRT in estimating premorbid intelligence, but extended the methodology by adding the Spot the Word Test (SWT) (Law and O'Carroll, 1998). The addition of a third index was prompted by the recognition that, in the face of increasingly severe dementia, even the CCRT underestimated scores. The NART and CCRT also share a limited effectiveness in the presence of aphasic and dysarthric patients, an additional factor that prompted the development of the SWT. In this paradigm, subjects are not required to read aloud, but must still make a lexical decision by indicating on a series of paired words which is the real and which is the pseudo word (Baddeley et al, 1993).

Comparing the three modalities in a sample of 21 elderly patients with Alzheimer's disease, 94 healthy volunteers and 20 patients with orthopedic injuries, results indicated that, while all three measures, namely the NART, CCRT and the SWT were relatively unaffected by dementia, only the NART and CCRT correlated well with current verbal intelligence. A final observation was that demented patients showed a significant improvement in performance compared to control subjects when the irregular words (i.e. NART items) were placed in contextual sentences. This led the authors to conclude that the CCRT was the preferred method of assessing premorbid intellect. A similar result has been found in a sample of 114 healthy subjects (Watt and O'Carroll, 1999).

Demographic variables
A number of demographic variables can be used to predict premorbid IQ. Variables such as education, occupation, race, age and gender are

introduced into a regression analysis to calculate the value of premorbid intellect, although results should be considered an approximation, not a precise estimate of IQ. For example, the Barona equation accounts for 38%, 24% and 36% of the vIQ, pIQ and full-scale IQ scores, respectively (Barona et al, 1984). From these figures it can be seen that demographic indices are better predictors of premorbid verbal as opposed to performance IQ. Other investigators have, however, derived equations that produced more robust results. Thus, Wilson's equation (Wilson et al, 1978) predicted 54% of the variance, while Crawford et al (1989b) were able to predict 50% of the variance in the full-scale WAIS IQ.

There are both advantages and disadvantages to this approach. On the plus side, the procedure is completely independent of the subject's current cognitive functioning. However, in some developmental disorders, including schizophrenia, the early onset of the morbid process may adversely affect the level of education and skill of the occupation, thereby influencing calculation-based estimates of premorbid intellect. In addition, even when these factors are not relevant to the subject, the regression analyses cannot furnish more than 50% of the variance scores. Estimates become particularly suspect when premorbid IQ lies at the extreme end of the normal IQ range, i.e. scores below 69 or greater than 120 (Barona et al, 1984; Sweet et al, 1990). Thus, demographic-based estimates should not be used in the gifted or the mentally retarded subject.

Evidence suggests that the NART and NAART are better predictors than demographic variables of verbal premorbid and full-scale IQ (Blair and Spreen, 1989).

WAIS subscales

Some of the subscales of the WAIS are more resistant to decay in acquired brain injury. Two verbal modalities (vocabulary and information) and one performance modality (picture completion) are considered best in this regard. Another view, allied to this, is that the WAIS should be completed and the highest score on a particular index taken as the marker of premorbid functioning and the standard by which current functioning should be judged (Lezak, 1983).

Combining measures

It makes intuitive sense that, if the NART and demographic variables both measure premorbid IQ, combining them may improve the accuracy of the measure. On balance, the data support this view, although not all studies are in agreement. There is evidence that adding demographic data to the NART increases the explained variance between 7 and 18%, depending on the study quoted (Crawford et al, 1989b; Watt and O'Carroll, 1999; Willshire et al, 1991). Two North American studies refuted this result (Blair and Spreen, 1989; Grober and Sliwinski, 1991). There are also data to show that demographic variables enhance the CCRT and the SWT as well (Watt and O'Carroll, 1999).

Conclusion

From a clinical point of view, the NART (or NAART) is easy to administer, takes no more than a few minutes to complete and is simple to score. While there is a tendency for scores to be underestimated in certain conditions, it provides a good approximation of premorbid intellectual abilities and places current cognitive performance in perspective. The Cambridge Contextual Reading Test is also relatively simple and quick to administer and, while there is considerably less published literature on this method compared to that of the NART, the test is to be preferred in the case of those disorders, such as moderate to severe dementia and early onset, institutionalized schizophrenia, where the validity of the NART is compromised. In research settings, the adjunctive use of demographic predictors enhances the accuracy of the assessment. All the measures mentioned in this chapter are in the public domain.

References

Austin M-P, Ross M, Murray C, O'Carroll RE, Ebmeier KP et al (1992) Cognitive function in major depression. *J Affect Disord* **25**:21–30.

Baddeley A, Emslie H, Nimmo-Smith I (1993) The spot-the-word test: a robust estimate of verbal intelligence based on lexical decision. *Br J Clin Psychol* **32**:55–65.

Barona A, Reynolds CR, Chastain R (1984) A demographically based index of pre-morbid intelligence for the WAIS-R. *J Consult Clin Psychol* **52**:885–887.

Beardsall L (1998) Development of the Cambridge Contextual Reading Test for improving the estimation of premorbid verbal intelligence in older persons with dementia. *Br J Clin Psychol* **37**:229–240.

Beardsall L, Brayne C (1990) Estimation of verbal intelligence in an elderly community: A prediction analysis using a shortened NART. *Br J Clin Psychol* **29**:83–90.

Beardsall L, Huppert FA (1994) Improvement in NART word reading in demented and normal older persons using the Cambridge contextual reading test. *J Clin Exp Neuropsychol* **16**:232–242.

Blackmore L, Crawford JR, Simpson SA (1994) Current and premorbid intelligence in Huntington's disease. *Proc Br Psychol Soc* **2**:57.

Blair JR, Spreen O (1989) Predicting premorbid IQ: A revision of the National Adult Reading Test. *Clin Neuropsychol* **3**:129–136.

Brayne C, Beardsall L (1990) Estimation of verbal intelligence in an elderly community: An epidemiological study using the NART. *Br J Clin Psychol* **29**:217–223.

Cockburn J, Keene J, Hope T, Smith P (2000) Progressive decline in NART score with increasing dementia severity. *J Clin Exp Neuropsychol* **22**:508–517.

Crawford JR, Besson JAO, Parker DM, Sutherland KM, Keen PL (1987) Estimation of premorbid intellectual status in depression. *Br J Clin Psychol* **26**:313–314.

Crawford JR, Besson JAO, Parker DM (1988) Estimation of premorbid intelligence in organic conditions. *Br J Psychiatry* **153**:178–181.

Crawford JR, Stewart LE, Besson JAO, Parker DM, De Lacey G (1989a) Prediction of WAIS IQ with the National Adult Reading Test: Cross-validation and extension. *Br J Clin Psychol* **28**:267–273.

Crawford JR, Stewart LE, Cochrane RHB, Foulds JA, Besson JA et al (1989b) Estimating premorbid IQ from demographic variables: regression equations derived from a UK sample. *Br J Clin Psychol* **28**:275–278.

Crawford JR, Parker DM, Allan KM, Jack AM, Morrison FM (1991) The Short NART: Cross-validation, relationship to IQ and some practical considerations. *Br J Clin Psychol* **30**:223–229.

Crawford JR, Besson JAO, Bremner M, Ebmeier KP, Cochrane RH et al (1992) Estimation of premorbid intelligence in schizophrenia. *Br J Psychiatry* **161**:69–74.

Cummings JL, Houlihan JP, Hill MA (1986) The pattern of reading deterioration in dementia of the Alzheimer type: observations and implications. *Brain Lang* **29**:315–323.

Dunkley G, Rogers D (1994) The cognitive impairment of severe psychiatric illness: a clinical study. In David AS, Cutting JC (eds) *The Neuropsychology of Schizophrenia*. Hove, UK: Lawrence Erlbaum Associates, 1994:181–196.

Ebmeier KP, Booker K, Cull A, Gregor A, Goodwin GM et al (1993) The validity of the National Adult Reading Test in estimating premorbid intellectual ability in long-term survivors of hemispheric glioma and whole brain irradiation – a pilot study. *Psychooncology* **2**:133–137.

Feinstein A, Brown R, Ron M (1994) Effects of practice of serial tests of attention in healthy subjects. *J Clin Exp Neuropsychol* **16**:436–447.

Folstein MF, Folstein SE, McHugh PR (1975) 'Mini-Mental State': A practical method for grading the cognitive state of patients for the clinician. *J Psychiatr Res* **12**:189–198.

Fromm D, Holland AL, Nebes RD, Oakley MA (1991) A longitudinal study of word-reading ability in Alzheimer's disease: Evidence from the National Adult Reading Test. *Cortex* **27**:367–376.

Grober E, Sliwinski M (1991) Development and validation of a model for estimating premorbid verbal intelligence in the elderly. *J Clin Exp Neuropsychol* **13**:933–949.

Hart S, Smith CM, Swash M (1986) Assessing intellectual deterioration. *Br J Clin Psychol* **25**:119–124.

Jacobson RR, Acker CF, Lishman WA (1990) Patterns of neuropsychological deficit in alcoholic Korsakoff's syndrome. *Psychol Med* **20**:321–334.

Jones P, Guth C, Lewis S, Murray R (1994) Low intelligence and poor educational achievement precede early onset schizophrenic psychosis. In David AS, Cutting JC (eds) *The Neuropsychology of Schizophrenia*. Hove, UK: Lawrence Erlbaum Associates, 131–144.

Joyce EM, Robbins TW (1991) Frontal lobe function in Korsakoff and non-Korsakoff alcoholics in planning and spatial working memory. *Neuropsychologia* **29**:709–723.

Kopelman MD (1989) Remote and autobiographical memory, temporal context memory and frontal atrophy in Korsakoff and Alzheimer patients. *Neuropsychologia* **27**:437–460.

Kopelman M (1991) Frontal dysfunction and memory deficits in the Alcoholic Korsakoff syndrome and Alzheimer-type dementia. *Brain* **114**:117–137.

Law R, O'Carroll RE (1998) A comparison of three measures of estimating premorbid intellectual level in dementia of the Alzheimer type. *Int J Geriatr Psychiatry* **13**:727–730.

Leng NRC, Parkin AJ (1988) Double dissociation of frontal dysfunction in organic amnesia. *Br J Clin Psychol* **27**:359–362.

Lezak MD (1983) *Neuropsychological Assessment*, 2nd Edn. New York: Oxford University Press.

Mayes AR, Mendell PR, MacDonald C (1991) Disproportionate intentional spatial-memory impairments in amnesia. *Neuropsychologia* **29**:771–784.

Nebes RD, Martin DC, Horn LC (1984) Sparing of semantic memory in Alzheimer's disease. *J Abnorm Psychol* **93**:321–330.

Nelson HE (1982) *National Adult Reading Test (NART): Test Manual*. Windsor, UK: NFER Nelson.

Nelson HE, McKenna P (1975) The use of current reading ability in the assessment of dementia. *Br J Clin Psychol* **14**:259–267.

Nelson HE, O'Connell A (1978) Dementia: the estimation of premorbid intelligence levels using the new adult reading test. *Cortex* **14**:234–244.

Nelson HE, Willison J (1991) *National Adult Reading Test (NART): Test Manual*, 2nd Edn. Windsor, UK: NFER Nelson.

O'Carroll RE, Gilleard CJ (1986) Estimation of premorbid intelligence in dementia. *Br J Clin Psychol* **25**:157–158.

O'Carroll RE, Baikie EM, Whittick JE (1987) Does the National Adult Reading Test hold in dementia? *Br J Clin Psychol* **26**:315–316.

O'Carroll RE, Moffoot A, Ebmeier KP, Goodwin GM (1992a) Estimating premorbid intellectual ability in the Alcoholic Korsakoff Syndrome. *Psychol Med* 22:903–909.

O'Carroll RE, Walker M, Dunan J, Murray C, Blackwood D et al (1992b) Selecting controls for schizophrenia research studies: the use of the National Adult Reading Test (NART) as a measure of pre-morbid ability. *Schizophr Res* 8:137–141.

O'Carroll RE, Curran SM, Ross M, Murray C, Riddle W et al (1994) The differentiation of major depression from dementia of the Alzheimer-type using within-subject neuropsychological discrepancy analysis. *Br J Clin Psychol* 33:23–32.

O'Carroll RE, Prentice N, Murray C, van Beck M, Ebmeier KP et al (1995) Further evidence that reading ability is not preserved in Alzheimer's disease. *Br J Psychiatry* 167:659–662.

Paque L, Warrington EK (1995) A longitudinal study of reading ability in patients suffering from dementia. *J Int Neuropsychol Soc* 1:517–524.

Patterson K, Graham N, Hodges JR (1994) Reading in dementia of the Alzheimer type: A preserved ability? *Neuropsychology* 8:395–407.

Raven JC (1958) *Mill Hill Vocabulary Scales*, 2nd edn London: HK Lewis.

Raven JC (1996) *Progressive Matrices: A Perceptual Test of Intelligence. Individual Form*. Oxford: Oxford Psychologists Press.

Shoqeirat MA, Mayes AR (1991) Disproportionate incidental spatial-memory and recall deficits in amnesia. *Neuropsychologia* 29:749–769.

Shoqeirat MA, Mayes A, MacDonald C, Meudell P, Pickering A (1990) Performance on tests sensitive to frontal lobe lesions by patients with organic amnesia: Leng and Parkin revisited. *Br J Clin Psychol* 29:401–408.

Spreen O, Strauss E (1998) *A Compendium of Neuropsychological Tests*. 2nd edn New York: Oxford University Press.

Sweet J, Moberg P, Tovian S (1990) Evaluation of Wechsler Adult Intelligence Scale-Revised premorbid IQ clinical formulas in clinical populations. *Psychol Assess* 2:41–44.

Watt KJ, O'Carroll RE (1999) Evaluating methods for estimating premorbid intellectual ability in closed head injury. *J Neurol Neurosurg Psychiatry* 66:474–479.

Wechsler D (1981) *Wechsler Adult Intelligence Scale-Revised*. New York: Psychological Corporation.

Wilkinson GS (1993) *WRAT3 Administration Manual*. Delaware: Wide Range.

Willshire D, Kinsella G, Prior M (1991) Estimating WAIS-R IQ from the National Adult Reading Test: A cross-validation. *J Clin Exp Neuropsychol* 13:204–216.

Wilson RS, Rosenbaum G, Brown G, Rourke D, Whitman D et al (1978) An index of premorbid intelligence. *J Consult Clin Psychol* 46:1554–1555.

chapter 3

Mini Mental State Examination

History of the development of the MMSE

On revisiting the original publication of the Mini Mental State Examination (MMSE) (Folstein et al, 1975), Alistair Burns aptly described his feelings as 'akin to a sense of awe' (Burns, 1998). Nowhere in psychiatric practice has there been a standardized instrument so widely used around the world. As of this writing, the MMSE has been cited on 13 000 occasions! It crosses every continent, culture and language (Appendix 3.1). Moreover, it has become the lingua franca of cognitive assessment. Clinicians naturally ask, 'What is the MMSE score?' in order to have a measure of cognitive function.

The MMSE is generally grouped into seven categories representing different cognitive domains or functions: orientation to time (5 points); orientation to place (5 points); registration of three words (3 points); attention and calculation (5 points); recall of three words (3 points); language (8 points); and visual spatial ability (1 point). Orientation, short-term memory and language skills clearly predominate in the MMSE.

Ironically, as Marshall Folstein the prime developer of the MMSE pointed out, its design was rather casual, deriving its component parts from items that were selected from various sources that Folstein could recall from his mentors and from textbooks he had read (Folstein, 1998). The main criterion for selection was that items could be applied 'without additional equipment at the bedside'. This simple feature appears to have been the key to its phenomenal usage. In the 1970s, clinicians were gaining awareness of the importance of assessing cognitive function in elderly patients. The MMSE came along at a time when the need was great, and yet no other instrument had captured the clinical marketplace. Perhaps it was the name 'Mini Mental State' that was attractive. Perhaps it was the fact that it tested a number of different cognitive domains, and not simply orientation and short-term memory. Its validity was assessed using the Wechsler Adult Intelligence Scale (WAIS) with Pearson R correlation of 0.78 for verbal intelligence quotient (IQ) and 0.66 for performance IQ. Excellent inter-rater and test–retest reliability was also demonstrated.

Its appeal to psychiatric residents is especially great. Residents yearn for standardized methods that require little critical thinking. The MMSE gives them such a methodology for assessing cognition in the clinical setting. This scale seems to find a middle ground measuring more than most basic areas, but also one which could be administered quickly and acceptably (Brayne, 1998). Compared to the detailed and cumbersome neuropsychological test batteries of the mid-1970s, the MMSE is considered brief and generally takes about 10 minutes to administer.

However, a number of limitations emerged with its widespread clinical usage (Brayne, 1998). Ceiling effects became obvious in younger, more intact individuals, while severely impaired patients showed marked floor effects. Many authors have highlighted the influence and bias of education (Magni et al, 1995), culture (Bohnstedt et al, 1994) and sensory impairment (Folstein et al, 1985). In response to many of the concerns about bias and vulnerability of administration, a standardized MMSE was subsequently developed to improve inter-rater reliability (Molloy et al, 1991). Others expanded the MMSE in order to make it more informative (Teng and Chui, 1987). These attempts will be described elsewhere, but the original MMSE with all its flaws and limitations has proved to be extremely robust and appears to be the assessment instrument of choice for clinicians around the world.

The multiple uses of the MMSE have been detailed (Brayne, 1998). These include clinical applications (Galasko et al, 1995), use in clinical research (Chui et al, 1994), correlation with imaging studies (Obara et al,

1994) and studying community populations (Brayne and Calloway, 1990; Jorm et al, 1994). The MMSE has been used as the core cognitive measure in a number of major epidemiological studies and instruments including the Diagnostic Interview Schedule (DIS) used by the National Institute of Mental Health (NIMH), the Epidemiologic Catchment Area (ECA) study in the United States (Farmer et al, 1995), the Canadian Study on Health and Aging (CSHA) and the Medical Research Council Cognitive Function and Ageing Study in the United Kingdom. While the test is not considered ideal by any measure, Brayne (1998) pinpointed its particular value: 'A shorter scale would never have been useful in such a variety of settings and longer cognitive testing is not acceptable to the populations being studied. It is simple and easily applied'.

A generation of clinicians seeking an acceptable and valid cognitive screening test appears to have been imprinted (like Lorenz' ducklings) on the MMSE and in all likelihood will continue to follow it for the foreseeable future. Brayne (1998) predicted 'heavy quotation' of the MMSE for another decade, but it appears that she may have sold short this feisty instrument.

Analyses and modifications of the MMSE

Before documenting the intense scrutiny to which the MMSE has been subjected and examining various recommendations for its improvement, let us review what Marshall Folstein himself said about its use after more than two decades of experience (Folstein, 1998). According to him, the score should be the raw number of correct answers (out of a total of 30 points). He criticizes the practice of changing the total for various reasons such as sensory impairment. Moreover, while there may be a natural inclination to make the test easy for patients, he argues that its score should be reported, as in the rest of clinical medicine, by simply recording observations before making any interpretations. Folstein (1998) noted many of the limitations of the MMSE for specific populations, such as those with focal brain disease. Sensitivity is limited for conditions involving frontal and subcortical changes, as occur in Pick's disease (frontotemporal dementia) (Axelrod et al, 1992), multiple sclerosis (Rao et al, 1991), Parkinson's disease and more recent experience with AIDS dementia. Folstein (1998) readily acknowledged the improvement in detection of such frontal/subcortical conditions by adding executive function tests (Royall et al, 1994). Specifically, Folstein highlighted the difference in difficulty between serial 7's and spelling WORLD backwards. He favors the practice of using the more difficult serial 7's, unless the patient refuses to try or is unable to perform the test at all. Others suggest WORLD backwards as the standard to be used (Molloy and Standish, 1997; Tombaugh and McIntyre, 1992).

Folstein also noted the problems in translation of the MMSE into other languages. Items such as 'no ifs, ands or buts' are designed as a 'series of short words of low probability of occurring together in a sentence'. Yet this phrase clearly favors native English speakers who recognize its idiomatic usage. Does spelling 'MONDO' backwards in Italian carry the same difficulty as 'WORLD'?

To his credit, Folstein is fully prepared to abandon the MMSE for what he calls a 'Micro Mental' test that may enhance the psychometric properties of a short cognitive screening instrument that is still 'practical, acceptable and sensitive at the bedside'. His willingness and openness to 'move on', however, is not yet shared by the world population of clinicians, who continue to hang on to the MMSE as an old, familiar friend who they are unwilling to abandon.

One cannot emphasize enough that the MMSE score is not a diagnosis, but as Folstein himself noted, it is 'merely a dimension of cognitive impairment'. Different brain syndromes may show specific patterns of impairment on the MMSE, but this is a matter of interpretation and analysis, and is in no way reflected by the score alone.

The standardized MMSE

Molloy and Standish (1997) addressed problems in the administration and scoring of the MMSE, as the original publication (Folstein et al, 1975) provided little direction. It left too much discretion to individual raters, who developed their own idiosyncratic practices such as awarding half points for some answers, giving hints and encouraging the subject during the test. The problem was particularly highlighted in multi-site clinical trials, where a great deal of time and effort was spent attempting to develop a consensus on how the MMSE should be administered and scored (Molloy and Standish, 1997).

Setting up

In setting up for the assessment, raters are asked to ensure that hearing or visual aids are in use. Raters are instructed that questions may be asked up to three times, and no clues or feedback are to be given during the test. Finally, some props are required including a large piece of paper with intersecting pentagons on one side and the instruction 'Close your eyes' on the other side. A sharpened pencil with an eraser is required and a watch or a clock is necessary to time each item. The standardized MMSE (SMMSE) also provides verbatim instructions for scoring each item. For orientation to time, leeway and consideration are given for a date that is 1 day before or after the actual date. Furthermore, special consideration is given on the first or last day of the month, or the first or last week of the season.

In order to decrease variability, the SMMSE exposes explicit time limits on all tasks; however, the subject is unaware of the timing in order not to influence performance. Specific instructions are provided for dealing with time issues in order to preserve the patient's dignity and avoid upsetting the patient, and thereby influencing the results.

Orientation to place: items are asked in order from the largest unit (e.g. country) to the smallest (e.g. floor). Depending on the unique circumstances of each place or building, a list of acceptable responses is generated.

The three-word registration and memory tasks are also standardized. The original MMSE used 'apple, penny and table'. However, alternative three-word sets are necessary when the MMSE is used repeatedly, thus avoiding a practice effect. Examples of other sets with similar word frequency are 'ball, car, man' and 'bull, war, pan'.

Attention and concentration are measured by two alternative tasks, namely the spelling of WORLD backwards and serial 7's, the latter being more difficult. For the WORLD task, the subject is first asked to spell WORLD forward. If the subject is unable to do this successfully, the score is zero. There are many possible combinations of errors for spelling WORLD backwards, and the SMMSE provides such a list with corresponding scores. Many centers test only the WORLD task for an elderly population.

Naming of 'watch and pencil' is very rigorously scored. Approximate answers such as 'clock' and 'pen' are not accepted.

The three-stage command is also a curiosity based on the original design of Folstein et al (1975). The SMMSE provides the following specific instruction: 'Take this paper in your (non-dominant) hand, fold the paper in half once with both hands, and put the paper down on the floor'. One may still ask why it is necessary to place the paper on the floor. Such bending poses potential orthopedic risks for both subject and rater alike (Figure 3.1).

Sentence completion must involve a subject, verb and object to score a point. Spelling mistakes are not penalized.

In the copy design task involving intersecting pentagons, a score of 1 point is awarded only if a four-sided figure is created by the overlap of the two pentagons. Irregularities created by hand tremor should not be penalized.

When comparing the SMMSE to the MMSE, the authors were able to demonstrate significant improvements in intra- and inter-rater variance and interclass correlation. Similarly, the mean time of administration was reduced from 13.39 minutes for the MMSE to 10.47 minutes for the SMMSE ($p < 0.004$).

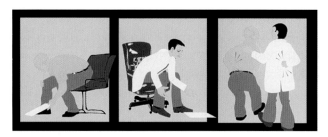

Figure 3.1 *Orthopedic hazards of the MMSE.*

Despite the obvious advantages of standardized administration of the MMSE, it is our experience that, more than 10 years after its original publication (Molloy et al, 1991), the SMMSE is not used routinely in the clinical setting. The durability of the original MMSE with its inherent weaknesses continues to impress.

The comprehensive review of the MMSE by Tombaugh and McIntyre

Readers are referred to a comprehensive review of the MMSE (Tombaugh and McIntyre, 1992). This paper is the most widely cited analysis of the psychometric properties and utility of the MMSE. They review variability in administration and scoring of the MMSE, as well as its reliability, validity, sensitivity and specificity.

Studies involving the full range of cognitive impairment in a variety of settings were reviewed. The main outcome measures against which the validity of the MMSE was assessed included 'gold standards' such as clinical diagnosis, the Diagnostic and Statistical Manual of the American Psychiatric Association (DSM-III-R), and the National Institute of Neurological and Communicative Disorders and Stroke-Alzheimer's Disease and Related Disorders Association (NINCDS-ADRDA) criteria. Longitudinal studies of dementia support the MMSE's construct validity, as scores generally decline between 2 and 5 points per year in such subjects.

Analyses of individual items
For both normal and demented subjects, analyses of the seven cognitive domains of the MMSE revealed that most of the errors occurred in four of the domains: recall of three words, attention and concentration (WORLD/serial 7's); pentagons; and orientation to time. This is similar to the findings on telephone cognitive screens (Jarvenpaa et al, 2002). Thus, the different items on the MMSE are not equally sensitive to severity of cognitive impairment. The WORLD/serial 7's domain shows marked differences. Spelling WORLD backwards produces higher scores than serial 7's and correlates better with the total MMSE score (Holzer

et al, 1984). Thus, WORLD should be the preferred choice for this item.

While concluding that the MMSE has largely fulfilled its goal of assessing severity of cognitive impairment and change over time, Tombaugh and McIntyre (1992) cite significant residual concerns. The first is the MMSE's lack of sensitivity to mild cognitive impairment and its failure to discriminate subjects with mild dementia from normal. Of course, the MMSE is not alone amongst screening instruments in this particular limitation. Clock-drawing has similar limitations (Powlishta et al, 2002). Furthermore, the MMSE's relative loading on verbal skills (versus visual spatial/constructional or executive functions) limits its utility in those individuals suffering from focal lesions to the right hemisphere, as well as subjects with primarily frontal deficits. The MMSE (like all cognitive screening tests) is not diagnostic, and abnormal scores simply indicate the need for further evaluation. Iverson (1998) suggests the following guidelines to determine when more comprehensive evaluation is necessary following a positive screening assessment with the MMSE. The first situation involves a score below the adjusted cut-off as well as corroborative evidence of cognitive impairment by history (usually through an informant). The second situation occurs when the individual score on retest exceeds the 0.95 confidence interval for possible measurement error (usually a decline of three points or more).

Modified MMSE

Another attempt to deal with the psychometric limitations of the MMSE and its lack of standardization was the development of the modified Mini Mental State (3MS) by Teng and Chui (1987). They added four items to the instrument: date and place of birth; animal naming; similarities; and a second recall task. This broadened the range and difficulty of cognitive testing. For finer discrimination, they increased the scoring range up to 100 points and produced a detailed manual for scoring and administration. Because the 3MS requires more time to administer and score, it must offer significantly superior validity (McDowell et al, 1997).

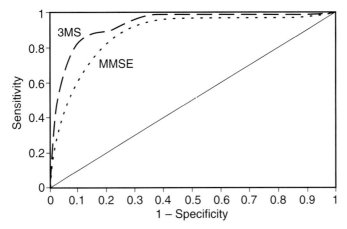

Figure 3.2   *3MS vs MMSE ROC curves. (Reproduced from McDowell et al, 1997, with permission from Elsevier Science.)*

In the CSHA, the 3MS was superior to the MMSE in sensitivity and specificity, reflected by areas under the receiver operating characteristic (ROC) curves (Figure 3.2).

Despite the superiority of psychometric properties demonstrated by the 3MS, once again our experience suggests that it has not been widely accepted in the clinical domain, long after its publication in 1987. Cognitive screeners appear to be voting with their feet and remain immutably resistant to changing established practices.

Age- and education-correlated cut-off scores

Education has been repeatedly shown to influence MMSE scores, and hence represents a potential source of bias leading to misclassification. Several cross-sectional studies have shown that the level of education affects both sensitivity and specificity. Some authors have suggested that 8 years or less of education carries a clear potential for misclassification. Moreover, education may not represent a psychometric bias alone, but is also associated with a variety of biological risk factors including smoking, hypertension, obesity and hypercholesterolemia. Therefore, education has also been considered an etiological risk factor for dementia.

Table 3.1 MMSE abnormal cut-off scores and reliable change difference scores (from Iverson, 1998, with permission from John Wiley & Sons Ltd).

Age/education (years)	n	Abnormal cut-off score	0.90	0.95	Reliable change difference score
60–64 years old					
0–4	88	19	1.46	1.74	2
5–8	310	22	1.77	2.12	3
9–12	626	25	1.30	1.55	2
13+	270	26	0.98	1.18	2
Total	1294	24	1.54	1.84	2
65–69 years old					
0–4	126	18	1.46	1.74	2
5–8	633	23	1.30	1.55	2
9–12	814	25	1.07	1.27	2
13+	358	27	0.77	0.92	1
Total	1931	24	1.23	1.47	2
70–74 years old					
0–4	139	19	1.30	1.55	2
5–8	533	23	1.38	1.65	2
9–12	550	24	1.23	1.47	2
13+	255	25	1.23	1.47	2
Total	1477	24	1.38	1.65	2
75–79 years old					
0–4	112	17	1.54	1.84	2
5–8	437	21	1.61	1.92	2
9–12	315	24	1.61	1.39	2
13+	181	25	1.23	1.47	2
Total	1045	22	1.61	1.92	2
80–84 years old					
0–4	105	16	1.69	2.02	3
5–8	241	21	1.46	1.74	2
9–12	163	21	1.77	2.12	3
13+	96	25	0.69	0.82	1
Total	605	21	1.69	2.02	3

Table 3.1 Continued

Age/education (years)	n	Abnormal cut-off score	0.90	0.95	Reliable change difference score
85+ years old					
0–4	61	14	2.23	2.67	3
5–8	134	17	2.52	3.02	4
9–12	99	22	1.54	1.84	2
13+	52	24	0.98	1.18	2
Total	346	19	2.23	2.67	3

These advanced interpretative data for the 'Field Survey form' of the MMSE were derived from data presented in the population forms (Crum et al, 1993). The Field Survey was published as an appendix by Folstein et al (1985). The abnormal cut-off scores are greater than 1.64 standard deviations below the sample means. The reliable change difference scores are calculated by multiplying the estimated standard error of difference score by a z-score of 1.64 or 1.96.

The widely accepted cut-off score for significant cognitive impairment has been less than 24/30 on the MMSE. However, this is less appropriate for the very old and those with limited education (Iverson, 1998). Table 3.1 provides guidelines for cut-off scores utilizing age and education as independent variables. Similarly, Bravo and Hebert (1997) provided scatter plots of average test scores versus age and education (Figure 3.3).

Summary

The MMSE has been subjected to a great deal of analysis and has been found wanting on several fronts. Nonetheless, it remains a core component of cognitive assessment worldwide and continues to be used in clinical research. Despite its clear limitations, its resilience and persistence in the clinical arena for over 25 years make it a truly historical instrument. As long as clinicians do not confer more weight than is

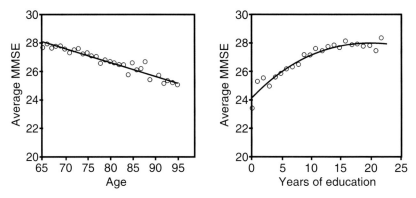

Figure 3.3 *Effect of age and education on MMSE scores. (Reproduced from Bravo and Hebert, 1997, with permission from John Wiley & Sons Ltd.)*

warranted to the MMSE score, its function remains useful as a signal that more evaluation and investigations are necessary or as a measure of change in cognitive status. Clinicians must still exercise their own executive function in the proper interpretation of the MMSE score. Moreover, they must still take a full history, consult informants and conduct appropriate auxiliary investigations. It is the clinician not the instrument that is responsible for any misuse or false interpretation of the MMSE score.

References

Axelrod BN, Goldman RS, Henry RR (1992) Sensitivity of the Mini-Mental State Examination to frontal lobe dysfunction in normal aging. *J Clin Psychol* **48(1)**:68–71.

Bohnstedt M, Fox PJ, Kohatsu ND (1994) Correlates of Mini-Mental State Examination scores among elderly demented patients: The influence of race–ethnicity. *J Clin Epidemiol* **47**:1381–1387.

Bravo G, Hebert R (1997) Age- and education-specific reference values for the Mini-Mental and modified Mini-Mental State Examinations derived from a non-demented elderly population. *Int J Geriatr Psychiatry* **12**:1008–1018.

Brayne C (1998) The Mini-Mental State Examination, will we be using it in 2001? *Int J Geriatr Psychiatry* **13**:285–294.

Brayne C, Calloway P (1990) The case identification of dementia in the community: A comparison of methods. *Int J Geriatr Psychiatry* **5**:309–316.

Burns A (1998) Mini-Mental State: A practical method for grading the cognitive state of patients for the clinician. *Int J Geriatr Psychiatry* **13**:285–294.

Chui HC, Lyness SA, Sobel E, Schneider LA (1994) Extrapyramidal signs and psychiatric symptoms predict faster decline in Alzheimer's disease. *Arch Neurol* **51**:676–681.

Crum RM, Anthony JC, Bassett SS et al (1993) Population-based norm for the Mini-Mental State Examination by age and education level. *JAMA* **269**:2386–2391.

Farmer ME, Kittner SJ, Rae DS (1995) Education and change in cognitive function: The Epidemiologic Catchment Area Study. *Ann Epidemiol* **5**:79–84.

Folstein M (1998) Mini-Mental and son. *Int J Geriatr Psychiatry* **13**:285–294.

Folstein M, Folstein S, McHugh P (1975) 'Mini-Mental State': a practical method for grading the cognitive state of patients for the clinician. *J Psychiatr Res* **12**:189–198.

Folstein M, Anthony JC, Parhad I, Duffy B, Gruenberg EM (1985) The meaning of cognitive impairment in the elderly. *J Am Geriatr Soc* **33**:228–235.

Galasko D, Edland SD, Morris JC, Clark C, Mohs R et al (1995) The Consortium to Establish a Registry for Alzheimer's Disease (CERAD) Part XI. Clinical milestones in patients with Alzheimer's disease followed over 3 years. *Neurology* **45**:1451–1455.

Holzer CE, Tischler GL, Leaf PJ et al (1984) An epidemiologic assessment of cognitive impairment in a community population. In: Greenley ED (ed) *Research in Community and Mental Health*. Greenwich: JAI Press, 3–32.

Iverson GL (1998) Interpretation of Mini-Mental State Examination scores in community-dwelling elderly and geriatric neuropsychiatry patients. *Int J Geriatr Psychiatry* **13**:661–666.

Jarvenpaa T, Rinne JO, Raiha I, Koskenvuo M, Lopponen M et al (2002) Characteristics of two telephone screens for cognitive impairment. *Dement Geriatr Cogn Disord* **13**:149–155.

Jorm AF, Christensen H, Henderson AS, Korten AE, Mackinnon AJ et al (1994) Complaints of cognitive decline in the elderly: A comparison of reports by subjects and informants in a community survey. *Psychol Med* **24**:365–374.

Magni E, Binetti G, Cappa S, Bianchetti A, Trabucchi M (1995) Effect of age and education on performance on the Mini-Mental State Examination in a healthy older population and during the course of Alzheimer's disease. *J Am Geriatr Soc* **43**:942–943.

McDowell I, Kristjansson B, Hill GB, Hébert R (1997) Community screening for dementia: The Mini Mental State Exam (MMSE) and modified Mini-Mental State Exam (3MS) compared. *J Clin Epidemiol* **50(4)**: 377–383.

Molloy DW, Standish TIM (1997) Mental status and neuropsychological assessment. A guide to the Standardized Mini-Mental State Examiniation. *Inter Psychogeriatr* **9(Suppl.1)**:87–94.

Molloy DW, Alemayehu E, Roberts R (1991) Reliability of a Standardized Mini-Mental State Examination compared with the traditional Mini-Mental State Examination. *Am J Psychiatry* **148(10)**:102–105.

Obara K, Meyer JS, Mortel KF, Muramatsu K (1994) Cognitive declines correlate with decreased cortical volume and perfusion in dementia of Alzheimer type. *J Neurol Sci* **127**:96–102.

Powlishta KK, Von Dra DD, Stanford A, Carr DB, Tsering C et al (2002) The clock drawing test is a poor screen for very mild dementia. *Neurology* **59**:898–903.

Rao SM, Leo GJ, Bernardin L, Unverzagt F (1991) Cognitive dysfunction in multiple sclerosis. 1. Frequency patterns, and prediction. *Neurology* **41**:685–691.

Royall DR, Mahurin RK, Cornell J (1994) Bedside assessment of frontal degeneration: distinguishing Alzheimer's disease from non-Alzheimer's cortical dementia. *Exp Aging Res* **20(2)**:95–103.

Teng EL, Chui HC (1987) The modified Mini-Mental State (3MS) Examination. *J Clin Psychiatry* **48**:314–318.

Tombaugh TN, McIntyre NJ (1992) The Mini-Mental State Examination: a comprehensive review [see comments]. *J Am Geriatr Soc* **40(9)**:922–935.

Appendix 3.1

Mini-Mental State Examination (MMSE)

The MMSE is organized in 5 sections:

			Maximum Score
1.	ORIENTATION	time and place	10
2.	REGISTRATION	3 objects	3
3.	ATTENTION & CALCULATION		
		serial 7's or spelling WORLD backwards	5
4.	RECALL	3 objects	3
5.	LANGUAGE	naming; repetition; 3-stage command; read and obey; sentence; copy design	9
		Total maximum score	30

chapter 4

The Clock Drawing Test

Clock drawing was recognized for many years as a component of cognitive assessment. Its origins can be traced to neurology journals which reported use of this test as a measure of parietal and hence visuospatial functioning (Critchley, 1966). Over the past 20 years, however, it has been used increasingly as a screening instrument for dementia and a wide range of neuropsychiatric disorders. Beginning with Goodglass and Kaplan (1983) clock drawing was incorporated into the Boston Asphasia Battery. Since then, there have been multiple studies in the literature addressing the screening function and psychometric properties of the clock drawing test including international reviews from Poland (Krzyminski, 1995); Israel (Heinik, 1998); Germany (Ploenes et al, 1994); Sweden (Agrell and Dehlin, 1998); China (Lam et al, 1998) and Japan (Nagahama et al, 2001). Over a dozen different scoring systems have been published since 1983 (Shulman, 2000).

*Cognitive and methodological issues

The need for a wide range of intellectual and perceptual skills to complete a task makes for a good cognitive screening instrument. Moreover, the many cognitive skills necessary for completion of the clock drawing

* Adapted with permission from Shulman (2000) *International Journal of Geriatric Psychiatry.*

test can be observed or inferred (Mendez et al, 1992; Royall et al, 1998) and include the following:

1. Comprehension (auditory)
2. Planning
3. Visual memory and reconstruction in a graphic image
4. Visuospatial abilities
5. Motor programming and execution
6. Numerical knowledge
7. Abstract thinking (semantic instruction)
8. Inhibition of the tendency to be pulled by perceptual features of the stimulus (i.e. the 'frontal pull' of the hands to '10' in the instruction 'ten past eleven')
9. Concentration and frustration tolerance

A mix of visuospatial abilities as well as executive control functions makes clock drawing particularly useful but also challenging in terms of scoring and interpretation (Royall et al, 1998).

The scoring systems described here are not all comparable because of differing emphasis on visuospatial, executive, quantitative and especially qualitative issues (Kaplan, 1990). Each scoring system uses slightly different methodologies and instructions for clock drawing. However, a consensus appears to be emerging towards a standardized approach. Most studies use a pre-drawn circle of approximately 4 inches (10 cm) in diameter. However, some authors still feel that there is value in observing subjects perform free-drawn circles (Freedman et al, 1994). Generally, the instructions to the patient are: 'This circle represents a clock face. Please put in the numbers so that it looks like a clock and then set the time to 10 minutes past 11'. This involves the abstract task of denoting time in symbolic fashion using hands and the tester should not use the word 'hands' in the instructions. While other times such as 3:00, 8:05 and 2:45 have been used, the 11:10 task is particularly useful because it includes both visual fields and also invokes the inhibition of the 'frontal pull' towards ten, an error commonly seen in mildly impaired subjects. The term 'clock drawing

Table 4.1 Psychometric properties of the clock drawing test (reproduced from Shulman, 2000, with permission from John Wiley & Sons Ltd).

Studies	Scoring systems	n	Specificity (%)	PPV (%)	NPV (%)	IRR	TRR	Correlation with other tests
Original scoring systems								
Death et al (1993)	4 classes	117	87	71	90			
Fujii et al (1998)	N/A	N/A	90					
Lam et al (1998)	10 points	53	79	98		0.94		Blessed DRS = 0.60 *MMSE (Chinese) = −0.65
Manos and Wu (1994)	10 points	97				0.92 (mean) (0.88–0.96)	(0.90) (mean) (0.87–0.94)	Block Design = 0.56 MMSE = 0.49 Trails A = 0.48
Mendez et al (1992)	20 points	46				0.94	0.78	Rey Complex Figure = 0.66 Symbol Digit = 0.65 MMSE = 0.45 GDS = 0.40

Table 4.1 Continued

Studies	Scoring systems	n	Specificity (%)	PPV (%)	NPV (%)	IRR	TRR	Correlation with other tests
Shua-Haim et al (1997)	6 points	88						MMSE = 0.57 Sunderland = 0.91
Shulman (2000)	5 points	75	72			0.75		*MMSE = −0.65 *SMSQ = −0.66
Shulman (2000) modified	6 points	183				0.96 (mean) (0.94–0.97)		*MMSE = −0.77 *GDS = −0.32
Sunderland et al (1989)	10 points							GDS = 0.56 DRS = 0.59 SPMSQ = 0.59 Blessed DRS = 0.51
Todd et al (1995)	10 points	23	92			0.96		
Tuokko et al (1992)	Qualitative errors >2	58	86			0.92 (mean) (0.90–0.95)	0.7	

Table 4.1 Continued

Studies	Scoring systems	n	Specificity (%)	PPV (%)	NPV (%)	IRR	TRR	Correlation with other tests
Watson et al (1993)	4 quadrants e4	76	82			0.93	0.63	
Wolf-Klein et al (1989)	10 patterns	325	93					
Replication studies								
Ben-Yehuda et al (1995)	Mendez	71	94	65	85			MMSE = 0.76
Bourke and Castleden (1995)	Mendez (M)	77				0.97		CAMCOG = 0.67 (M)
	Shulman (S)					0.91		CAMCOG = 0.70 (S)
	Pentagon					0.98		MMSE = 0.58 (M)
								MMSE = 0.56 (S)
Brodaty and Moore (1997)	Shulman (12)	28	86	96		0.89		MMSE = 0.62
	Sunderland		79	83		0.92		MMSE = 0.73
	Wolf-Klein		79	89		0.88		MMSE = 0.58
Dastoor et al (1991)	Shulman (11)	102						*HDS = −0.38

Table 4.1 Continued

Studies	Scoring systems	n	Specificity (%)	PPV (%)	NPV (%)	IRR	TRR	Correlation with other tests
Gruber et al (1997)	Wolf-Klein	145	75	79	42	94		SPMSQ = 0.40
Huntzinger et al (1992)	Sunderland	431						OMCT = 0.30
Libon et al (1993)	Sunderland (modified)	64						Wechsler Memory = 0.33
								Trails A = −0.34
								Go-No-Go = 0.37
								Bloc design = 0.42
								Hooper visual = 0.37

* Negative correlation reflects the scoring system used for the clock test.

DRS, Dementia Rating Scale; GDS, Global Deterioration Scale; HDS, Hierarchic Dementia Scale; MMSE, Mini-Mental State Examination; OMCT, Orientation-Memory-Concentration Test; SMSQ, Short Mental Status Questionnaire; SPMSQ, Short Portable Mental Status Questionnaire; PPV, positive predictive value; NPV, negative predictive value; IRR, inter-rater reliability; TRR, test–retest reliability.

test' is used to include those scoring systems that also involve clock setting and clock reading.

Table 4.1 summarizes the main psychometric properties of each screening test. A brief summary of the highlights of each published scoring system is provided below. The mean sensitivity and specificity are each 85%. Most studies used the Diagnostic and Statistical Manual of the American Psychiatric Association (DSM-III-R) and the National Institute of Neurological and Communicative Disorders and Stroke-Alzheimer's Disease and Related Disorders Association (NINCDS-ADRDA) criteria as the gold standard, although a few used clinical diagnosis. Readers are referred to the original references for further details. Figures 4.1 and 4.2 provide examples of typical qualitative errors and Figure 4.3 indicates the clinical usefulness of clock drawing in demonstrating cognitive change. Characteristic errors include perseveration; right–left confusion; concrete thinking, especially the tendency to 'pull' the minute hand towards '10'; and confusion about the concept of time.

Original scoring systems

In perhaps its first systematic use, Goodglass and Kaplan (1983) included the clock test as part of the Boston aphasia battery. The procedure involves clock setting where the subject is given four pre-drawn clock faces including short lines marked in the positions of the 12 numbers. The subject is then asked to denote four different times: 1:00, 3:00, 9:15 and 7:30. One point is awarded for each correct placement of a hand and one point each for correctly drawing the relative lengths of the minute and hour hand. Three points can be achieved for each clock for a maximum of 12 points on the test. Age and level of education appear to be influential factors in only those scoring in the bottom range.

Shulman et al (1986) compared the clock drawing test to the Mini Mental State Examination (MMSE) (Folstein et al, 1975) and the Short Mental Status Questionnaire (SMSQ) (Robertson et al, 1982). The mean age of the 75 subjects was 75.5 years. Three groups included those with

Severity
 Score

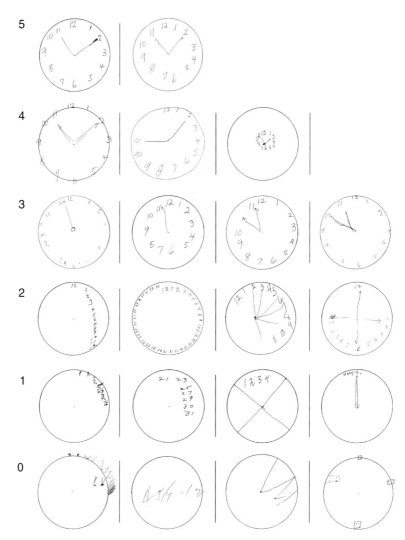

Figure 4.1   *Severity scores from 5 to 0. (Reproduced from Shulman, 2000, with permission from John Wiley & Sons Ltd.)*

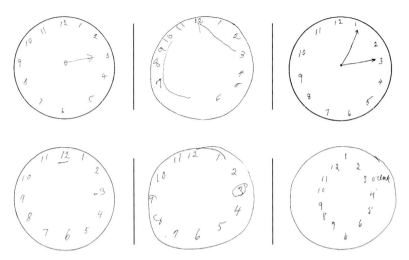

Figure 4.2 *Errors in denoting 3 o'clock. (Reproduced from Shulman, 2000, with permission from John Wiley & Sons Ltd.)*

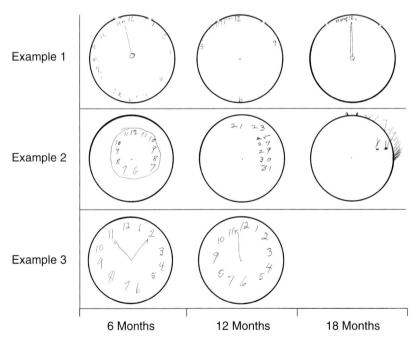

Figure 4.3 *Sensitivity to deterioration in dementia. (Reproduced from Shulman, 2000, with permission from John Wiley & Sons Ltd.)*

dementia, those with depression and normal controls. A five-point scale of severity of impairment was developed, based on clinical experience. A score of 1 denoted subtle errors while a score of 5 was given when the subject was unable to make any reasonable attempt to draw a clock. In a later study (Shulman et al, 1993) this five-level scoring system was modified to reverse the order, giving the highest score to an intact clock and the lowest to the most impaired. Our current practice (Figure 4.1) is to give 5 points for a 'perfect' clock. A score of 4 is given for minor visuo-spatial errors; 3 for inaccurate representation of 10 past 11 when the visuospatial organization is well done; 2 for moderate visuospatial disor-ganization of numbers such that accurate denotation of 'ten past eleven' is impossible; 1 for a severe level of visuospatial disorganization; and zero for inability to make any reasonable representation of a clock.

Sunderland et al (1989), using a priori criteria, developed a 10-point scale with 10 as the best score and 1 as the worst score. Five points are given for drawing a clock face with circle and numbers intact, while 6–10 points are assigned for accuracy of drawing hands to denote the time 2:45. An arbitrary cut-off score of 6 out of 10 is considered within normal limits. Three out of 83 controls (3.6%) scored less than 6, whereas 15 out of 67 of Alzheimer's patients (22.4%) scored more than 6 (Fisher's exact test, $p < 0.001$).

Wolf-Klein et al (1989) tested consecutive outpatients who were screened for cognitive impairment. They compared their clock test to the MMSE, Hachinski's scale (Hachinski et al, 1974) and the Dementia Rating Scale (Blessed et al, 1968). Using a pre-drawn circle, ten hierarchi-cal clock patterns were predetermined by a previous pilot study involv-ing over 300 patients. The diagnostic categories of their patients included normals, those with Alzheimer dementias and multi-infarct dementias, and others. A cut-off score of 7–10 reflected a normal response and an 'abnormal' score was less than 7. With a focus on tem-poroparietal function, they found that scores of 1–6 were specific for Alzheimer's disease as opposed to multi-infarct dementia or mixed cases.

Tuokko et al (1992) use a procedure which involves three empirically derived tasks including clock drawing, clock setting and clock reading. Clock drawing involved a pre-drawn circle in which the subject is asked to denote 'ten past eleven'. Clock setting involves five different times and clock reading involves the same clocks as in clock setting but in a different order. Errors on clock drawing are classified according to the following categories: omissions, perseverations, rotations, misplacements, distortions, substitutions and additions. Clock setting achieves a maximum of 3 points (adapted from Goodglass and Kaplan, 1983). Clock reading also achieves a maximum of 3 points. More than two errors was considered a positive (abnormal) result for clock drawing, while the cut-off for the clock setting and clock reading tasks was a score of less than 13. Four error categories (omissions, distortions, misplacements and additions) contributed significantly to the difference between normal elderly and Alzheimer's disease patients.

Mendez et al (1992) described the Clock Drawing Interpretation Scale (CDIS) tested on patients with dementia. Their scoring system includes: general impression, 3 points; 'code number' items, 12 points; 'code hands' items, 5 points; total, 20. All normal subjects scored 18 or more on the CDIS while 8.7% of Alzheimer's disease patients scored 18 or more.

Fujii (1992) developed theoretically based scoring criteria for the clock drawing test with high sensitivity and specificity. In a subsequent report (Fujii et al, 1998) the clock drawing tests were scored according to their criteria and the authors found the clock drawing test to be better than the MMSE at detecting milder cases of dementia.

Death et al (1993) focused on cognitive screening of elderly in-patients, both medical and surgical. Their scoring system includes four classes: 1, bizarre; 2, major spacing problems; 3, minor spacing problems; 4, completely normal. Only classes 3 and 4 are considered to be within normal limits.

The 'clock completion' test (Watson et al, 1993) includes a pre-drawn circle and the subject is asked to draw in the numbers on a clock face but not asked to draw the hands on the clock. Analysis included only the positioning of the clock numbers. The scoring system divided the pre-drawn circle into four quadrants with greatest weighting given to the fourth quadrant. Any error in quadrants one to three received a score of 1; any error in quadrant four received a score of 4. A score of

0–3 was considered normal and anything ≥ 4 was considered abnormal (i.e. suffering from dementia). They studied a group of patients from a geriatric outpatient assessment clinic and found an excellent comparison with the Blessed Orientation-Memory-Concentration test.

The '10-point clock test' (Manos and Wu, 1994) includes a scoring system that utilizes a transparent circle divided into eighths applied to the clock drawn by the patient. Points are given for the numbers falling into their proper segment as well as points given for hands correctly drawn, to a maximum of ten. Some significant errors will not be scored by this method. These include the counter clockwise placement of numbers or numbers placed outside the circle. An arbitrary cut-off score of 7 out of 10 points identified 76% of patients diagnosed with dementia and 78% of the control patients. Other scoring systems tested, including that of Mendez et al (1992) (cut-off 18/20), identified 90% of Alzheimer patients and 100% of controls. Tuokko et al (1992) (cut-off at more than two errors) identified 86% of Alzheimer patients and 92% of controls; while Sunderland et al (1989) (cut-off 6/10) identified 78% of Alzheimer's disease patients and 96% of controls. In a cautionary note regarding the interpretation of tests reported in the literature, they observed that the more impaired the dementia sample and the less impaired the controls the better the discrimination by any screening test.

The normative study of clock drawing (Freedman et al, 1994) proposes an empirically derived test based on clinical interpretation as well as the 'process' oriented approach of Kaplan (1990). A scoring system is provided for a normative population in seven different age ranges from 20 to 90 years. Their study involves five test administration conditions:

1. A free drawn condition with a requirement to draw all aspects of the clock including 15 'critical' items and time setting for 6:45
2. A pre-drawn clock set to 6:05 including 13 'critical' items
3. Three different 'examiner' clocks denoting 11:10, 8:20 and 3:00 o'clock.

Because of the length and complexity of the scoring system, it appears best suited for research purposes.

Todd et al (1995) studied a somewhat atypical population consisting of a relatively small sample of patients with dementia. The mean age was only 58 years for the dementia group as opposed to 67 years for the normal population. There were significant differences in education for the dementia population (8 versus 12 years for normal controls). No specific instructions for clock drawing were given except for the time instruction of 8:05. The scoring system was derived from the scoring procedure of the Rey complex figure test (Taylor, 1959). Five categories were included: shape; numbers 1–6; numbers 7–12; short arm; and long arm. Given the small numbers and the rather atypical population (i.e. younger and less educated), the impressive psychometric properties reported in the study need to be viewed with some caution, because of the question of generalizability.

Shua Haim et al (1997) performed a retrospective chart analysis of patients with a mean age of 77 years in an outpatient memory disorders clinic. They utilized a simple scoring system (SSS) with a maximum of 6 points. The scoring is based largely on the visuospatial aspects of the task and the correct denotation of time by the hands of the clock. A formula was developed using simple linear regression that related clock scores with the MMSE as follows: MMSE = 2.4 × (the clock score) + 12.7. A clock score of zero on the SSS predicts an MMSE score of < 13, whereas a clock score equal to a maximum of 6 predicts an MMSE score of ≥ 27.

Replication studies

Dastoor et al (1991) found a good correlation between the clock drawing test (Shulman et al, 1986) and the Hierarchic Dementia Scale (Cole and Dastoor, 1983). This dementia scale, although well validated, has not been used in any of the other studies reported in this review. Using these tests, the authors were able to differentiate a group of elderly depressives from dementing subjects.

Huntzinger et al (1992) screened randomly selected medical–surgical outpatients using the clock drawing scoring system of Sunderland et al (1989). They compared clock dawing to the six-item Orientation-

Memory-Concentration Test (OMCT) (Katzman et al, 1983). Clock drawing scores of 8–10 were considered to reflect mild impairment or normal functioning; a score of 5–7 represented moderate impairment; and a score less than 5 indicated severe impairment. The OMCT did not identify 7% of patients who had moderate to severe impairment on clock drawing. Unfortunately, the OMCT is not as widely used as the MMSE for comparison purposes.

Libon et al (1993) focused on the addition of a copy condition to the command instruction for the clock drawing test according to Sunderland et al (1989). The 'copy' condition places no demands on auditory comprehension or visual memory but the subject must have visuospatial ability and execute the drawing in a planned and organized fashion. The authors attempted to differentiate Alzheimer's disease from cerebrovascular disease. They examined the utility of the copy condition in 34 Alzheimer's disease subjects and 30 cerebrovascular subjects who had consecutive admissions to the Philadelphia Geriatric Center Consultation and Diagnostic Program. Normal controls were community dwelling and were recruited from an Active Life Program. In the copy condition, the Alzheimer's disease patients did significantly better than the cerebrovascular disease patients. Only the Alzheimer's disease group significantly improved from the command to the copy condition. The authors concluded that the clock drawing test may differentiate the dementia patients from normals and that the copy condition may expand the clinical usefulness of the test by differentiating subtypes of dementia. This study was limited by the relatively small number of patients with Alzheimer's disease (n = 34) and cerebrovascular disease (n = 30), and therefore will require replication.

Bourke and Castleden (1995) compared the clock drawing test (Mendez et al, 1992; Shulman et al, 1993) and the pentagon test of the MMSE and correlated these tests with the full MMSE and the CAMCOG (Roth et al, 1986). Emphasis was placed on the need to score the hand placements on the clock drawing test. False negatives occurred in 43% on the Mendez scale; 17% on the Shulman scale and 36% on the pentagons.

Ben-Yehuda et al (1995) used the CDIS of Mendez et al (1992) and compared it to the MMSE in a sample of hospitalized elderly patients admitted via the emergency department. The authors considered the clock drawing test to be an effective cognitive screening test that was 'psychologically non-threatening'. The low specificity of the study may have been due to the relatively low cut-off score used for normals with the MMSE.

Gruber et al (1997) compared the clock drawing test (Wolf-Klein et al, 1989) to the Short Portable Mental Status Questionnaire (SPMSQ) (Pfeiffer, 1975) in consecutive outpatients in a geriatric psychiatry clinic at the University of Texas. A significant limitation of this study was the fact that only the SPMSQ score was used as a criterion for the presence or absence of cognitive impairment, hence the kappa score was only 0.4. The presence of psychiatric illness may have accounted for the poor correlation and low sensitivity and specificity.

Brodaty and Moore (1997) studied consecutive referrals to a memory disorders clinic. They compared three scoring systems: the modified system of Shulman et al (1993); that of Sunderland et al (1989); and that of Wolf-Klein et al (1989). In support of Tuokko et al (1992), they concluded that spacing errors may be a particularly good discriminator of normal versus abnormal cognition. They also noted that time setting seems to increase the test's sensitivity. With regard to false negatives (those patients with a working diagnosis of dementia who scored 'normal' on the MMSE), the scale of Shulman et al (1993) identified 87.5% of that sample as impaired compared to 62.5% with Sunderland et al (1989) and Wolf-Klein et al (1989). This is a reflection of the specificity of each test. In the false-negative rate of normal clock test but abnormal MMSE, Shulman et al (1993) and Sunderland et al (1989) were equal at 15%, while the Wolf-Klein scale had a false-negative rate of 25%. They concluded that the clock test adds an assessment of frontal and temporo-parietal function to the cognitive screening process and recommend (like Stahelin et al, 1997) the MMSE plus the clock test to increase the sensitivity and specificity of the cognitive screening process.

Cultural, ethnic and linguistic considerations

Borson et al (1999) evaluated the clock drawing test alone without the memory task to determine its utility in a sample of individuals with a multicultural, multiethnic and diverse educational background. The clock drawing test was essentially similar in its ability to detect dementia to two longer screening instruments (the MMSE and the Cognitive Abilities Screening Instrument (CASI)). However for a poorly educated (fewer than 8 years of education) and non-English speaking group, the clock drawing test was able to identify probable dementia cases with a sensitivity of 94% and specificity of 85%, better than the other two screening instruments. Moreover, the clock drawing test had less information lost due to non-completion (8%) compared to the MMSE (12%) and CASI (16%).

Borson et al (2000) argued that telling of time by clock face is familiar in all major cultures and civilizations, whereas the more abstract figure copying (as in the MMSE intersecting pentagons) is a skill more familiar to those educated in developed countries.

The task of clock drawing 'from scratch' requires the use of multiple cognitive abilities from a wide range of cerebral regions. This is ideal for a cognitive screening instrument. However, this is not true of other screening and visuospatial copying tasks. This 'diffuse' task is therefore ideal for cognitive screening purposes. Borson et al (1999) list a number of the cognitive abilities elicited by the clock drawing test: long-term memory and information retrieval, auditory comprehension, visuospatial representation, visual perceptive and visual motor skills, global and hemispheric attention, simultaneous processing and, perhaps most important, executive functions (Royall, 2000).

Ainslie and Murden (1993) compared three scoring systems: those of Shulman et al (1986); Sunderland et al (1989) and Wolf-Klein et al (1989). They demonstrated the impact of low education on decreasing the specificity in the Shulman and Sunderland scales but not in the Wolf-Klein scale. However, the Wolf-Klein scale had an unacceptably low sensitivity of 48% in their sample. They concluded that clinicians must use caution in the use of the clock drawing test when subjects with low education are screened for dementia.

Silverstone et al (1993) reported on the usefulness of the clock drawing test in a group of 18 Russian immigrants who were unable to speak English. Screening with the clock drawing test identified four subjects with abnormal scores. Follow-up with these patients' families confirmed a diagnosis of progressive cognitive loss and dementia. The authors suggested that the clock drawing test may be useful where language is a serious barrier to cognitive testing.

Predictive validity

The predictive validity of the clock test was assessed using a longitudinal method in order to identify differences between subjects who were not demented and those who were in the early stages of a progressive dementia (O'Rourke et al, 1997). Fifty-nine subjects were assessed again if they had not met criteria for dementia at the initial assessment. The mean time between the initial and follow-up assessment was 22 months. At follow-up, 22 of these 59 individuals with a mean age of 64 were diagnosed with dementia at the second assessment using the NINCDS-ADRDA criteria. The clock test differentiated the group that eventually demented from that which remained normal, with a sensitivity of 91% and a specificity of 95%. The relatively small sample size invites replication of this study.

Lee et al (1996) studied the clock drawing test's ability to distinguish the early stages of Alzheimer's disease from normal aging. They studied 30 subjects using the NINCDS-ADRDA criteria. All patients had a clinical dementia rating score of 0.5 (questionable) to 2.0 (moderate severity). Only those patients were included who scored 0.5 on the Clinical Dementia Rating (CDR) scale (questionable dementia) and who went on to score at least 1.0 on the CDR follow-up. These individuals were considered very mild cases of dementia at the initial assessment, and went on to a progressive decline in cognition as measured by the CDR. The Sunderland and Mendez scoring systems were used as well as the MMSE. Nine patients out of the 30 had a CDR score of 0.5 at the initial assessment and declined in cognition. Only three out of these nine individuals scored less than 6 on the scale of Sunderland et al (1989) at baseline, thus yielding an apparent sensitivity of only 33%. The authors concluded that in very mild cases the clock drawing test had limited value.

However, it is important to note that none of the normals in their study had abnormal clock scores. In fact, a very good correlation was demonstrated between the mean clock scores and the mean CDR scores from normal to increasing severity, including a significant difference between the very mild cases (CDR = 0.5) and normal cases. This study needs to be replicated before concluding that the clock drawing test is not sensitive to very mild cases.

Shulman et al (1993) followed a large group of dementing individuals living in the community with their caregivers. In a study designed to predict survival in the community, the clock test proved to be extremely sensitive to cognitive decline in this group of dementing individuals on both quantitative and qualitative measures. Moreover, dementing individuals who had experienced a significantly greater decline on the clock test at 1-year and 2-year follow-ups were more likely to have caregivers who had decided to institutionalize them. It was hypothesized that the decision to institutionalize was based in part on the perception of a rapid decline in the cognitive function of their dependant as reflected by the change on the clock test itself. The authors concluded that the clock test appears to be a useful adjunct in monitoring change in individuals suffering from progressive dementia in the community.

Clock drawing and other neuropsychiatric conditions

Executive cognitive screening

Donald Royall and colleagues at the University of Texas Health Science Center in San Antonio have championed the notion that executive dysfunction is an early and sensitive marker for dementia. Royall (2000) notes that executive control function (ECF) was added by the American Psychiatric Association to its list of deficits in the diagnosis of dementia. Executive functions are defined as 'cognitive processes that orchestrate complex and goal-directed activities' (Royall, 2000). These executive deficits in turn may lead to behavioral difficulties, disorganization and ultimately decline in function. ECF is largely associated with the prefrontal cortex; however, ECF is also dependent on a well-integrated frontal subcortical system (Cummings, 1993).

Royall argues for two types of dementia (type 1 and type 2). ECF impairment is central to both types but in type 1 dementias there are clinical signs of posterior (temporal–parietal) cortical dysfunction. Type 2 dementias which primarily involve ECF include some potentially reversible conditions such as major depression, vascular disease and adult onset diabetes mellitus. Royall (2000) argues that type 2 presentations occur more commonly in the very old and may indeed comprise the majority of very late onset dementias as well as mild cognitive impairment seen in 'normal aging'. In light of the concern related to disorders that specifically affect frontal/executive function, Royall et al (1998) developed a variant of the clock drawing test (CLOX) designed to detect executive impairment and differentiate it from non-executive visuospatial failure.

Royall et al (1998) counter the misconception that clock drawing tests are primarily visuospatial tasks and therefore sensitive specifically to right parietal pathology. Other studies by the same group have found impairment on the clock drawing test in non-cortically impaired subjects (Royall and Polk, 1998).

CLOX: 'The executive clock drawing task'

This 'executive' test is divided into two parts in order to distinguish the executive control of clock drawing from the constructional/visuospatial ability. The executive functions relevant to the clock drawing test include goal selection, planning, motor sequencing, selective attention and self monitoring of a subject's current action plan. For the first part of the test (CLOX 1), the subject is instructed to draw a clock on blank paper with the following instruction: 'Draw me a clock that says 1:45. Set the hands and numbers on the face so that a child could read them'. The instructions can be repeated for clarity but no other assistance is offered. The detailed scoring system for CLOX 1 is appended (Appendix 4.1). The notion underlying the method for CLOX 1 is that it reflects performance in a novel and ambiguous situation eliciting the executive skills listed above. Some of the instructions are designed to deliberately

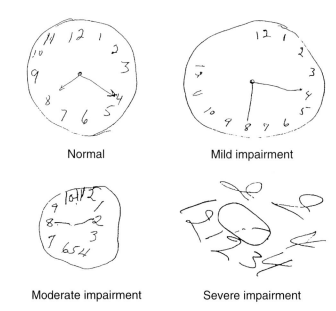

Normal   Mild impairment

Moderate impairment   Severe impairment

Figure 4.4 *CERAD scoring for CDT. (Reproduced from Borson et al, 1999, with permission from The Gerontological Society of America.)*

distract the subject. For example, the use of the terms 'hand' and 'face' may trigger semantic intrusions because they are more commonly associated with body parts than with elements of a clock. The number '45' may elicit a concrete response to the number itself or components '4 or 5'. The maximum CLOX score is 15.

CLOX 2 is a simple copying task of the pre-drawn clock already set at 1:45. Differences between CLOX 1 and 2 scores are hypothesized to reflect executive contribution to the clock drawing test versus constructional and visuospatial ability (Figure 4.5). Note that intersecting pentagons derived from the MMSE are essentially copying tasks and are not impaired in pure frontal dysfunction.

In Alzheimer's disease (Figure 4.5), the clock drawing test is impaired in both unprompted and copying tasks. Subject C in Figure 4.5 suffers from a vascular dementia without cortical features and hence only the unprompted clock drawing test is affected, i.e. copy task is intact. In subject A, an independent elderly control, the presence of an essential tremor does not seem to affect clock scores in a qualitative way.

CLOX Test

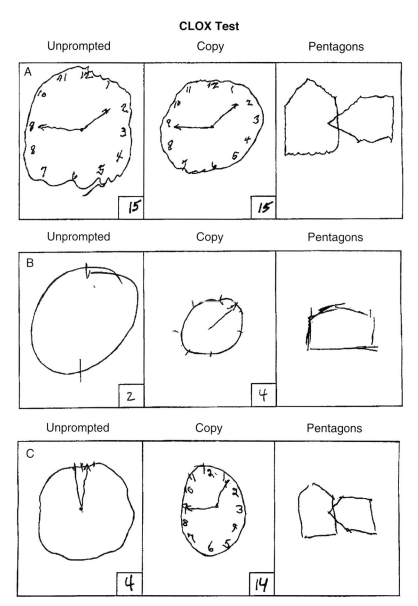

Figure 4.5 Qualitative differences in CLOX performance, in a normal elderly control, a patient with Alzheimer's disease, and a patient with non-cortical vascular disease. (A) An 82-year-old elderly control. EXIT25=08/50 (scores>5/50 impaired), MMSE=29/30 (scores<24/30 impaired). (B) A 74-year-old married white woman with Alzheimer's disease. EXIT25=21/50(24/50) comparable with six-year-old children or residents requiring skilled nursing), MMSE=12/30. (C) A 74-year-old right-handed white man with a history of coronary artery disease (status post myocardial infarction), hypertension, non-insulin dependent diabetes mellitus, and falls. EXIT22=24/50, MMSE=28/30. (Reproduced from Royall et al, 1998, with permission from the BMJ Publishing Group.)

The authors used Exit 25 as a measure of executive control (Royall et al, 1992). Scores on Exit 25 (0–50) correlate well with other measures of ECF including the Wisconsin Card Sort (r = 0.54) and trail-making part B (r = 0.64). Higher scores on Exit 25 are associated with greater impairment. The cut-off score of less than 15/50 best discriminates non-demented elderly controls. Since Exit 25 accounted for most of the variance in CLOX 1 (the executive component) scores, the authors suggested that this confirms construct validity. The pattern of CLOX 1/CLOX 2 scores correctly classified 91.9% of Alzheimer's disease subgroups with and without constructional impairment as measured by the MMSE pentagons. Royall et al (1998) concluded that the CLOX test may be able to distinguish clinically homogeneous groups with Alzheimer's disease or possibly distinguish Alzheimer dementias from non-Alzheimer cases.

In a comparison of CLOX to five other scoring methods for the clock drawing test, the CLOX test explained more variance in ECF than other clock drawing tests (Royall et al, 1999). Nonetheless, all clock drawing tests demonstrated significant correlation with Exit 25, that is executive function. However, none of the other tests specifically highlight the executive control function in their methodology or scoring. It appears that clock drawing tests represent 'a potentially easy, reliable and cost-effective means of measuring ECF' (Royall et al, 1999).

Delirium

Fisher and Flowerdew (1995) used the clock drawing test to predict post-operative delirium in older patients who were undergoing elective orthopedic surgery. While this study has yet to be replicated, it does represent a potential use of the clock drawing test. Elderly patients undergoing elective hip and knee surgery were examined pre- and postoperatively, using a modified Confusion Assessment Method (CAM) Questionnaire (Inouye et al, 1990). Using step-wise multiple logistic regression, they identified two significant risk factors for postoperative delirium. The first was male gender, but the second was a clock drawing score of ≤ 6 out of a possible 10 points, based on a modified clock drawing scoring system (Sunderland et al, 1989; Wolf-Klein et al, 1989). Overall, 17% of the patients developed a postoperative delirium (Table 4.2).

Table 4.2   Risk factors for postoperative delirium.

Patients with postoperative delirium	Odds Ratio
Males (11/37) (30%)	5.6 (1.9–33.8)
Clock score ≤ 6 (6/11) (55%)	9.0 (2.8–45.6)
Males with clock score ≤ 6 (5/6) (83%)	20.8 (4.1–1033)

(Adapted from Fisher and Flowerdew, 1995.)

Interestingly, an abnormal MMSE score did not predict delirium in this model. The authors speculated that the clock drawing test measures non-dominant parietal functions better than the MMSE, and therefore may be indirectly detecting an increased predisposition to the development of delirium. By identifying high-risk patients for delirium, one may be able to decrease the morbidity associated with delirium by timely interventions.

Manos (1998) reported a case in which the clock drawing test was used to document recovery from a delirium up to 14 days postoperatively. By postoperative day 10, the delirium had cleared from a clinical perspective, but cognitive impairment was still evident on the clock drawing test, with minor impairment noted up to day 14. This provides further evidence of the usefulness of clock drawing in monitoring the course of delirium.

Vascular dementia
Meier (1995) reported a unique strategy in the clock drawing task that appears to be more common in patients with vascular dementia. Specifically, this involves first dividing the circle with radial lines into segments. In a comparison of the frequency of segmentation patterns in clock drawings of patients with Alzheimer's disease compared to vascular dementia, the vascular patients used the strategy at twice the rate. Almost half of all impaired clock drawings of vascular dementia patients showed segmentation compared with only one-quarter of the impaired clock drawings of Alzheimer's patients. Moreover, patients using segmentation had a higher score on the MMSE than patients with other strategies.

Qualitative analyses of clock drawings were used in an attempt to demonstrate differences in the neuropsychological profiles of Alzheimer's disease compared to vascular dementia (Kitabayashi et al, 2001). Using the schema proposed by Rouleau et al (1992), they performed qualitative analyses on clock drawings and found Alzheimer's disease patients' error patterns to be stable and independent of severity. However, in patients with vascular dementia, there was evidence of increased frequency of graphic difficulties and conceptual deficits as the severity of the dementia worsened. However, the frequency of visuospatial or planning deficits decreased with dementia severity (Kitabayashi et al, 2001). In mild dementia, the frequency of spatial and planning deficits was lower in vascular dementia while, in the moderate dementia group, vascular dementia patients showed an increased frequency of graphic difficulties.

The finding of increased spatial and planning deficits in mild vascular dementia suggests that frontal–subcortical disturbances are operative. However, at the moderate stage, conceptual deficits and graphic difficulties become more frequent, while the spatial and conceptual deficits decrease, suggesting that the impairment of memory and motor function mask the frontal executive dysfunction as dementia severity increases.

The authors suggest that cognitive profiles are significantly different between Alzheimer's disease and vascular dementia at the mild and moderate levels and it may be possible to discriminate between these types of dementia by using qualitative analyses of clock drawings.

Heinik et al (2002) used CAMCOG-derived clock drawings to compare Alzheimer's patients with those suffering from vascular dementia. While there was no significant difference in the overall level of cognitive performance measured by the MMSE and CAMCOG, the total clock score based on the scoring system of Freedman et al (1994) did show a difference between the two groups. Only the total score and the hands subscore of Freedman et al (1994) differentiated the vascular dementia patients. The authors attributed this difference to a presumed sensitivity of the clock drawing test to executive dysfunction, which tends to be more pronounced in vascular dementia patients compared to those with Alzheimer's disease.

Roman and Royall (1999) make the case for using ECF as a mechanism underlying the diagnosis of vascular dementia and differentiating it from Alzheimer's disease. Royall (2000) have argued elsewhere that there are essentially two types of dementia. Type I dementias directly affect the posterior cortical association regions. Alzheimer's disease represents the most common form of this syndrome. In contrast, Type II dementia pathology is limited to the frontal systems and vascular dementia is a more common example of this type. The distinctive pattern of impairment on executive measures has been used to differentiate the two conditions (Roman and Royall, 1999). Hence, the CLOX test, which is an executive clock drawing test, may very well be useful in differentiating vascular dementia on this theoretical basis and based on the previous work of Royall (2000).

Stroke
Suhr et al (1998) examined the utility of the clock drawing test and localizing lesions resulting from various strokes. They hypothesized that the qualitative aspects of clock drawing would be more useful than quantitative measures in discriminating patients with respect to lesion location. The qualitative assessment was done according to the methodology proposed by Rouleau et al (1992) and described above. In comparing six different clock scoring methods, they found no significant difference between various lesion groups using quantitative scoring techniques in assessing localization of function. However, qualitative features did demonstrate the ability to differentiate between lesion groups. Specifically, right hemisphere stroke patients showed more graphic difficulties and impaired spatial planning compared to left hemisphere stroke patients. This is consistent with the impaired visuospatial/visuoconstructional difficulties seen after right hemisphere strokes. Furthermore, subcortical patients showed more graphic difficulties compared to cortical patients, while cortical patients demonstrated more perseveration on qualitative assessments. This is similar to the findings described by Rouleau et al (1992) with respect to the subcortical dementias associated with Huntington's disease, where graphic difficulties were more common.

Parkinson's disease

In the description of clock drawing in a variety of neurological disorders, Dal Pan et al (1989) studied three groups of patients: normal controls, those with probable Alzheimer's disease and non-demented Parkinson's disease patients. They used a clock drawing test with criteria that resulted in scores from a minimum of zero to a maximum of four. These criteria have not been validated, although subsequent studies of simplified scoring systems suggest that this approach is probably a valid method of measuring cognitive impairment.

Diffuse abnormalities on the clock drawing test were seen only in patients with Alzheimer's disease and other types of dementia. In contrast, non-demented Parkinson's disease patients showed a distinct pattern of abnormalities on clock drawing. Specifically, their errors were limited to spacing of numbers within the circle; abnormalities of perceptual motor co-ordination (including micrographia) as a result of poor planning, and monitoring of movement. Stern (1983) has postulated

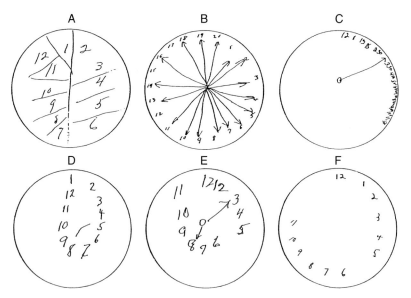

Figure 4.6 *Clock drawings in neurological disorders. A–C, Alzheimer's disease; D–F, Parkinson's disease. (Reproduced from Dan Pan et al, 1989, with permission from IOS Press.)*

that the basal ganglia play a role in planning and sequencing, as well as modulating behavior and may be responsible for the abnormalities seen in clock drawing. The author concluded that the clock drawing test identifies those with dementia syndrome, but not subtypes. Furthermore, clock drawing may distinguish non-demented Parkinson's disease patients from those with dementia, in particular in relation to the planning function (Figure 4.6).

White matter lesions

Skoog et al (1996) assessed the clock drawing test in both demented and non-demented 85-year-old patients with respect to white matter lesions. There was a significant interaction effect between white matter lesions and cerebral infarctions in this group of patients, resulting in a lowering of cognitive performance as measured by clock drawing. White matter lesions resulted in lower clock scores in both demented and non-demented 85-year-old patients.

Huntington's disease

Rouleau et al (1992) used both quantitative and qualitative analyses of clock drawings in an attempt to distinguish characteristics associated with Huntington's disease and Alzheimer's disease (Figures 4.7 and 4.8). The clock drawing test was adapted from the Boston Parietal Lobe Battery (Goodglass and Kaplan, 1983). They added a qualitative analysis which included: (a) graphic difficulties to stimulus-bound responses, e.g. for 11:10, hand pointing to the '10' rather than '2' (Figure 4.7) and for 1:45 the hands pointing to '4' and '5' (Figure 4.9); (b) conceptual deficits; (c) spatial or planning deficits; (d) perseveration.

This study included a copy task in which Alzheimer's patients showed significant improvement compared to Huntington's disease patients. The authors suggest that the drawing problems are not primarily due to graphic, motor or visual perceptual difficulties, but rather to the loss of semantic associations with the word 'clock'. Huntington's versus Alzheimer's patients demonstrated moderate to severe graphic and planning deficits. The planning deficits may be related to frontostriatal dysfunction associated with Huntington's disease. Since the overall level of

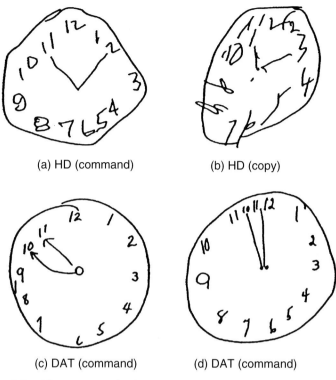

(a) HD (command)   (b) HD (copy)

(c) DAT (command)   (d) DAT (command)

Figure 4.7 *Visuoconstructive impairment in Huntington's disease (HD) and dementia of the Alzheimer type (DAT). Samples of errors observed. Graphic difficulties: (a) moderate, (b) severe. Stimulus-bound response: (c) associated with visuospatial deficit, (d) associated with a conceptual deficit in representing the time on the clock. (Reproduced from Rouleau et al, 1992, with permission from Elsevier Science.)*

cognitive impairment was equal between Alzheimer's and Huntington's patients, the qualitative differences noted above appear to be due to different involvement of the limbic cortical regions in Alzheimer's disease compared to the basal ganglia and corticostriatal dysfunction associated with Huntington's disease.

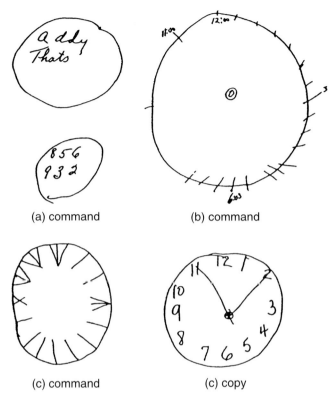

(a) command   (b) command

(c) command   (c) copy

Figure 4.8 *Visuoconstructive impairment in Alzheimer's dementia. (Reproduced from Rouleau et al, 1992, with permission from Elsevier Science.)*

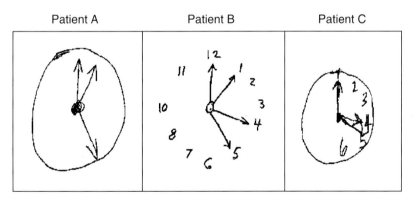

Figure 4.9 *Stimulus-bound errors in clock drawing (of time 1:45). (Reproduced from Royall et al, 1999, with permission from The Gerontological Society of America.)*

Discussion

Despite significant variations in the development of scoring systems that emphasize visuospatial and executive functions to different degrees, the psychometric properties of all the clock tests are remarkably consistent. Sensitivity and specificity levels are both at a mean of 85% for all published studies with excellent inter-rater reliability and good concurrent and predictive validity. Moreover, the clock drawing test appears to have achieved widespread clinical utilization, albeit with inconsistent approaches to scoring and interpretation. The literature reflects the interest and focus on this test in recent years, and conclusions are uniformly positive. The clock test appears to be, at the very least, an important adjunct to the cognitive screening process and very sensitive to cognitive change.

From a clinical perspective, the clock test provides an easy to use visual record of cognitive function that is appealing to busy clinicians. Generally, it takes less than a minute to conduct and score and appears to have achieved general acceptability on the part of patients. Clinical experience also indicates that it has had a tremendous effect on caregivers who are often shocked and surprised to see the extent of difficulty on this task performed by their impaired dependants. This has often helped to highlight the extent of the cognitive problem when caregivers are unaware or in denial. While there continues to be concern regarding the impact of education and language on the clock drawing test, it may be less pronounced than other instruments such as the MMSE that rely more heavily on language.

It is of interest that the clock drawing test, which appears to be so sensitive to cognitive decline in dementia, does not test recent memory, which has been considered the hallmark of dementing disorders. This suggests a reconsideration of the nature of the dementing process and just how the clock drawing test is able to reflect brain dysfunction without formally testing memory. Moreover, Royall et al (1998) who developed the 'CLOX' test, have added an important dimension to the interpretation of the clock drawing test, namely, its ability to tap into executive functions. This is a deficiency in most of the available simple cognitive screening tests and adds an aspect of the clock test that has been overshadowed by its obvious visuospatial focus. The 'process' approach of Kaplan (1990) also highlights the value of examining the qualitative aspects of clock drawing that inform our understanding of brain function.

In this chapter, the full range of published scoring systems have been presented, all of which seem to have excellent psychometric properties and all have similar conclusions regarding the use and value of the clock drawing test as a cognitive screening instrument. One should logically conclude from this that the simpler the scoring system the better. The more complicated and lengthy scoring systems do not appear to add significant value to the psychometric properties or clinical utility of this test. Ultimately, the clinical 'market place' should determine which scoring system has most practical value. However, the system used by the Consortium to Establish a Registry for Alzheimer's Disease (CERAD) seems optimal (Borson et al, 2000) (Figure 4.4, see p. 62).

Inevitably, the question of the impact of digital clocks arises. While it is difficult to predict the future use of analog clocks, it is safe to say that, for the current cohort of adults (40+), traditional clock drawing will remain a valid test for at least 30 years. If the clock test lasts that long, it will have outlived the usefulness of most tests in medicine.

As a single screening instrument, the clock drawing test clearly has limitations, as described by Borson et al (2000) in their testing of the Mini-Cog battery. Furthermore, in cases of very mild to mild dementia, the clock drawing test does appear to be limited, as do most single screening instruments (Lee et al, 1996; Powlishta et al, 2002; Storey et al, 2001). However, its very short administration time, simplicity and acceptability make its psychometric properties especially appealing. This also makes it a highly desirable item to include in a brief battery that aims to broaden its screening net, as in the Mini-Cog and GPCOG.

References

Agrell B, Dehlin O (1998) The clock-drawing test. *Age Ageing* 27:399–403.
Ainslie NK, Murden RA (1993) Effect of education on the clock-drawing dementia screen in non-demented elderly patients. *J Am Geriatr Soc* 41(3):249–252.

Ben-Yehuda A, Bentur N, Friedman G (1995) The clock drawing test as a cognitive screening tool for elderly patients in an acute-care hospital. *Aging* 7:188–190.

Blessed G, Tomlinson BE, Roth M (1968) The association between quantitative measures of dementia and of senile changes in the cerebral gray matter of elderly subjects. *Br J Psychiatry* **114**:797–811.

Borson S, Brush M, Gil E, Scanlan JM, Vitaliano PP et al (1999) The clock drawing test: utility for dementia detection in multi-ethnic elders. *J Gerontol Med Sci* **54A**:M534-M540.

Borson S, Scanlan J, Brush M, Vitaliano P, Dokmak A (2000) The Mini-Cog: A cognitive 'vital signs' measure for dementia screening in multi-lingual elderly. *Int J Geriatr Psychiatry* **15**:1021–1027.

Bourke J, Castleden CM (1995) A comparison of clock and pentagon drawing in Alzheimer's disease. *Int J Geriatr Psychiatry* **10**:703–705.

Brodaty H, Moore CM (1997) The clock drawing test for dementia of the Alzheimer's type: A comparison of three scoring methods in a memory disorders clinic. *Int J Geriatr Psychiatry* **12**:619–627.

Cole MG, Dastoor DP (1983) The Hierarchic Dementia Scale. *J Clin Exp Gerontol* **5**:219–234.

Critchley M (1966) *The Parietal Lobes*. New York: Hafner Publishing Company.

Cummings JL (1993) Frontal-subcortical circuits and human behavior. *Arch Neurol* **50**:873–880.

Dal Pan G, Stern Y, Sano M, Mayeux R (1989) Clock-drawing in neurological disorders. *Behav Neuro* **2**:39–48.

Dastoor DP, Schwartz G, Kurzman D (1991) Clock-drawing – An assessment technique in dementia. *J Clin Exp Gerontol* **13**:69–85.

Death J, Douglas A, Kenny RA (1993) Comparison of clock drawing with Mini Mental State Examination as a screening test in elderly acute hospital admissions. *Postgrad Med J* **69**:696–700.

Fisher BW, Flowerdew G (1995) A simple method for predicting postoperative delirium in older patients undergoing elective orthopedic surgery. *J Am Geriatr Soc* **43**:175–178.

Folstein M, Folstein F, McHugh PR (1975) Mini-Mental State: A practical guide for grading the cognitive state of patients for the clinician *J Psychiatr Res* **12**:189–198.

Freedman M, Leach L, Kaplan E, Winocur E, Shulman KI et al (1994) *Clock Drawing. A Neuropsychological Analysis*. Oxford: Oxford University Press.

Fujii DE (1992) The clock drawing test as a screening measure for dementia of the Alzheimer type: development and validation of a theoretically based scoring criteria. *Dissert Abst Int* **53(4-B)**: 2059.

Fujii DE, White L, Ross WG, Masaki KH, Petrovitch H et al (1998) A comparison of the clock drawing test and Mini Mental Status Examination screening for dementia in older-Japanese-American males in Hawaii. *Int Neuropsychol Soc* (abstract).

Goodglass H, Kaplan E *The Assessment of Aphasia and Related Disorders*. Philadelphia: Lea and Febiger.

Gruber NP, Varner RV, Chen Y-W, Lesser JM (1997) A comparison of the clock drawing test and the Pfeiffer Short Portable Mental Status Questionnaire in a geropsychiatry clinic. *Int J Geriatr Psychiatry* **12**:526–532.

Hachinski VC, Lassen NA, Marshall J (1974) Multi-infarct dementia: a cause of mental deterioration in the elderly. *Lancet* 2:207.

Heinik J (1998) Clock-drawing test in dementia due to Alzheimer's disease. *Harefuah* **134(2)**:143–148.

Heinik J, Solomesh I, Raikher B, Lin R (2002) Can clock drawing test help to differentiate between dementia of the Alzheimer's type and vascular dementia? A preliminary study. *Int J Geriatr Psychiatry* **17**: 699–703.

Huntzinger JA, Rosse RB, Schwartz BL, Ross LA, Deutsch SI (1992) Clock drawing in the screening assessment of cognitive impairment in an ambulatory care setting: A preliminary report. *Gen Hosp Psychiatry* **14(2)**:142–144.

Inouye SK, van Dyck CH, Alessi CA et al (1990) Clarifying confusion: The confusion assessment method. A new method for detection of delirium. *Ann Intern Med* **113**:941–948.

Kaplan E (1990) The process approach to neuropsychological assessment of psychiatric patients. *J Neuropsychiatry* **2**:72–87.

Katzman R, Brown T, Fuld P, Peck A, Schechter R et al (1983) Validation of a short orientation–memory concentration test of cognitive impairment. *Am J Psychiatry* **140**:734–739.

Kitabayashi Y, Ueda H, Narumoto J, Nakamura K, Kita H et al (2001) Qualitative analyses of clock drawings in Alzheimer's disease and vascular dementia. *Psychiatry Clin Neurosci* **55**:185 191.

Krzyminski S (1995) Test rysowania zegara. The clock-drawing test. *Postepy Psychiatrii I Neurologii* **1**:21–30.

Lam LWC, Chiu HFK, Ng KO, Chan C, Chan WF et al (1998) Clock-face drawing, reading and setting tests in the screening of dementia in Chinese adults. *J Gerontol* **53B**:352–357.

Lee H, Swanwick GRJ, Coen RF, Lawlor B (1996) Use of the clock drawing task in the diagnosis of mild and very mild Alzheimer's disease. *Int Psychogeriatr* **8**:469–476.

Libon DJ, Swenson RA, Barnoski EJ, Sands LP (1993) Clock drawing as an assessment tool for dementia. *Arch Clin Neuropsychol* **8**: 405–415.

Manos PJ (1998) Monitoring cognitive disturbance in delirium with the ten-point clock test. *Int J Geriatr Psychiatry* **13**:642–648.

Manos PJ, Wu R (1994) The ten point clock test: a quick screen and grading method for cognitive impairment in medical and surgical patients. *Int J Psych Med* **24**:229–244.

Meier D (1995) The segmented clock: a typical pattern in vascular dementia. *J Am Geriatr Soc* **43(9)**:1071–1073.

Mendez MF, Ala T, Underwood K (1992) Development of scoring criteria for the clock drawing task in Alzheimer's disease. *J Am Geriatr Soc* **40(11)**: 1095–1099.

Nagahama Y, Okina T, Nabatame H, Matsuda M, Murakami M et al (2001) Clock drawing in dementia: Its reliability and relation to the neuropsychological measures. *Clin Neurol* **41**:653–658.

O'Rourke N, Tuokko H, Hayden S, Beattie BL (1997) Early identification of dementia: Predictive validity of the clock test. *Arch Clin Neuropsychol* **12(3)**:257–267.

Pfeiffer E (1975) A short portable mental status questionnaire for the assessment of organic brain deficit in elderly patients. *J Am Geriatr Soc* **23**:433–441.

Ploenes C, Sharp S, Martin M (1994) The Clock Test: Drawing a clock for detection of cognitive disorders in geriatric patients [German]. *Zeitschrift Gerontol* **4**:246–252.

Powlishta KK, Dras V, Stanford A, Carr DB, Tsering C et al (2002) The clock drawing test is a poor screen for very mild dementia. *Neurology* **59**:898–903.

Robertson D, Rockwood K, Stolee P (1982) A Short Mental Status Questionnaire. *Can J Aging* **1**:16–20.

Roman GC, Royall DR (1999) Executive control function: A rational basis for the diagnosis of vascular dementia. *Alzheimer Dis Assoc Disord* **13**(3): S69-S80.

Roth M, Tyne E, Mountjoy Q, Huppert FA, Hendrie H et al (1986) CAMDEX: A standardized instrument for the diagnosis of mental disorder in the elderly with special reference to the early detection of dementia. *Br J Psychiatry* **149**:698–709.

Rouleau I, Salmon DP, Butters N, Kennedy C, McGuire K (1992) Quantitative and qualitative analyses of clock drawings in Alzheimer's and Huntington's disease. *Brain Cogn* **18**:70–87.

Royall DR (2000) Executive cognitive impairment: A novel perspective on dementia. *Neuroepidemiology* **19**:293–299.

Royall DR, Polk M (1998) Dementias that present with and without posterior cortical features: an important clinical distinction. *J Am Geriatr Soc* **46**:98–105.

Royall DR, Mahurin RK, Gray KF (1992) Bedside assessment of executive cognitive impairment: the executive interview. *J Am Geriatr Soc* **40**:1221–1226.

Royall DR, Cordes JA, Polk M (1998) CLOX: an executive clock drawing task. *J Neurol Neurosurg Psychiatry* **64**:588–594.

Royall DR, Mulroy A, Chiodo LK, Polk MJ (1999) Clock drawing is sensitive to executive control: a comparison of six methods. *J Gerontol Psych Sci* **54B**:P328–P333.

Shua-Haim J, Koppuzha G, Shua-Haim V, Gross J (1997) A simple scoring system for clock drawing in patients with Alzheimer's disease. *Am J Alzheimer's Dis* **September/October**:212–215.

Shulman KI (2000) Clock-drawing: Is it the ideal cognitive screening test? *Int J Geriatr Psychiatry* **15**:548–561.

Shulman KI, Shedletsky R, Silver IL (1986) The challenge of time: Clock-drawing and cognitive function in the elderly. *Int J Geriatr Psychiatry* **1**:135–140.

Shulman KI, Gold DP, Cohen CA, Zucchero C (1993) Clock-drawing and dementia in the community: A longitudinal study. *Int J Geriatr Psychiatry* **8**(6):487–496.

Silverstone FA, Duke WM, Wolf-Klein GP (1993) Clock drawing helps when communication fails [letter]. *J Am Geriatr Soc* **41**:1155.

Skoog IBS, Johansson B, Palmertz B, Andreasson LA (1996) The influence of white matter lesions on neuropsychological functioning in demented and non-demented 85-year-olds. *Acta Neurol Scand* **93**:142–148.

Stahelin HB, Monsch AV, Spiegel R (1997) Early diagnosis of dementia via a two-step screening and diagnostic procedure. *Int Psychogeriatr* **9**(Suppl. 1): 123–130.

Stern Y (1983) Behavior and the basal ganglia. In Mayeux R, Rosen WG (eds) *The Dementias, Advances in Neurology*, Volume 38. New York: Raven Press, 195–209.

Storey JE, Rowland JT, Basic D, Conforti DA (2001) A comparison of five clock scoring methods using ROC (receiver operating characteristic) curve analysis. *Int J Geriatr Psychiatry* **16**:394–399.

Suhr J, Grace J, Allen J, Nadler J, McKenna M (1998) Quantitative and qualitative performance of stroke versus normal elderly on six clock drawing systems. *Arch Clin Neuropsychol* **13**(6):495–502.

Sunderland T, Hill JL, Mellow AM, Lawlor BA, Gundersheimer BA et al (1989) Clock drawing in Alzheimer's disease: A novel measure of dementia severity. *J Am Geriatr Soc* **37**(8):725–729.

Taylor EM (1959) *The Appraisal of Children with Cerebral Deficits*. Cambridge, MA: Harvard University Press, 1959.

Todd ME, Dammers PM, Adams SG Jr, Todd AM, Morrison M (1995) An examination of a proposed scoring procedure for the clock drawing test: Reliability and predictive validity of the clock scoring system (CSS). *Am J Alzheimer's Dis* **July/August**:22–26.

Tuokko H, Hadjistavropoulos T, Miller JA, Beattie BL (1992) The clock test: A sensitive measure to differentiate normal elderly from those with Alzheimer Disease. *J Am Geriatr Soc* **40**(6):579–584.

Watson YI, Arfken CL, Birge SJ (1993) Clock completion: An objective screening test for dementia. *J Am Geriatr Soc* **41**(11): 1235–1240.

Wolf-Klein GP, Silverstone FA, Levy AP, Brod M (1989) Screening for Alzheimer's disease by clock drawing, *J Am Geriatr Soc* **37**(8):730–734.

Appendix 4.1 (reproduced from Royall, 1995, with permission from The BMJ Publishing Group)

CLOX: An Executive Clock Drawing Task©

STEP 1: Turn this form over on a light colored surface so that the circle below is visible. Have the subject draw a clock on the back. Instruct him or her to '**Draw me a clock that says 1:45. Set the hands and numbers on the face so that a child could read them.**' Repeat the instructions until they are clearly understood. Once the subject begins to draw no further assistance is allowed. Rate this clock (CLOX 1).

STEP 2: Return to this side and let the subject observe you draw a clock in the circle below. Place 12, 6, 3, and 9 first. Set the hands again to '1:45'. Make the hands into arrows. Invite the subject to copy your clock in the lower right corner. Score this clock (CLOX 2).

RATING			
Organizational Elements	*Point Value*	*CLOX 1*	*CLOX 2*
Does figure resemble a clock?	1		
Outer Circle Present	1		
Diameter > 1 inch?	1		
All numbers inside the circle?	1		
12, 6, 3, and 9 placed first?	1		
Spacing Intact? (Symmetry on either side of the 12–6 axis?) If 'yes' skip next.	2		
If spacing errors are present, are there signs of correction or erasure?	1		
Only Arabic numerals? 1			
Only numbers 1–12 among the Arabic numerals present?	1		
Sequence 1–12 intact? No omissions or intrusions.	1		
Only two hands present?	1		
All hands represented as arrows?	1		
Hour hand between 1 and 2 o'clock?	1		
Minute hand longer than hour?	1		
None of the following 1) hand pointing to 4 or 5 o'clock? 2) '1:45' present? 3) intrusion from 'hand' or 'face' present? 4) any letters, words or pictures? 5) any intrusion from circle below?	1 **TOTAL**		

chapter 5

Tests of frontal lobe function

In approaching the subject of frontal lobe tests, a brief overview of the anatomy of the frontal lobes is helpful. While prefrontal areas are of central importance in various aspects of cognitive functioning, additional motor and premotor areas also fall under the anatomical frontal rubric. This chapter, therefore, will briefly describe the anatomy and function of these areas. Thereafter, an approach to cognitive testing of frontal lobe functions based on the anatomical divisions will be delineated. A description of more complex, psychometric 'frontal' tests will be given, all of which are in the public domain and relatively straightforward to administer. Finally, a list of bedside, frontal tests will be provided and their validity discussed.

Frontal anatomy

The motor and premotor systems

The motor cortex (Brodmann area 4), lying anterior to the central sulcus, subserves motor tasks and is intricately involved in pyramidal function. It receives cortical projections from sensory parietal areas and subcortical connections from the thalamus. Efferent pathways traverse the internal capsule en route to the pyramidal tracts. Lesions in the motor cortex produce contralateral paralysis or paresis.

The premotor system (Brodmann 6) is important for integrating motor and sensory function and is thus connected to the primary sensory cortex, somatosensory cortex, primary motor cortex plus thalamus and extrapyramidal areas such as the caudate nucleus. Lesions in this area give rise to apraxia and difficulties with fine movement.

Frontal eye fields

This area (Brodmann 8) controls voluntary conjugate eye movement and is connected by long association bundles with other cortical regions, most prominently the occipital cortex and by projection fibers with the brain stem and oculomotor nerves. Lesions in the frontal eye fields will produce transient ipsilateral eye deviation and contralateral gaze paresis (Malloy and Richardson, 1994).

Broca's area

This corresponds to Brodmann area 44, in the lower frontal convolution. It is connected to areas in the prefrontal cortex (Brodmann 10) and supplementary motor areas. A lesion here produces a non-fluent speech disorder, characterized by effortful, grossly impaired expression and agrammatism, but intact comprehension.

The prefrontal cortex

The *dorsolateral prefrontal cortex* circuit begins at the lateral aspect of the frontal lobe and courses to the dorsolateral head of the caudate nucleus and then on to the globus pallidus and substantia nigra via direct and indirect pathways, relaying in the ventral anterior and medial dorsal nuclei of the thalamus before reconnecting to the dorsolateral prefrontal cortex.

The *ventral prefrontal circuit* originates in the inferior aspect of the prefrontal cortex and sequentially encompasses the ventromedial caudate nucleus, the globus pallidus, substantia nigra and subthalamic nuclei and finally the ventral anterior and medial dorsal thalamic nuclei prior to the circuit returning to the inferior prefrontal cortex. While this circuit and the dorsolateral prefrontal circuit share superficial similarities in terms of pathways, they relay with different sets of nuclei within the striatum and thalamus. Thus, they should be viewed as discrete, parallel circuits and it is this anatomical separation that dictates their very different clinical characteristics.

The third frontal subcortical circuit begins in the *anterior cingulate*, progresses to the ventral striatum, where it receives connections from limbic structures (such as the hippocampus, amygdala and entorhinal cortex) and sends connections to the globus pallidus and substantia nigra and then on to the medial dorsal nucleus of the thalamus, amongst other areas, before the circuit loops back to the anterior cingulate.

Lesions affecting this circuit produce varying degrees of apathy, ranging from poor motivation to the striking clinical picture of akinetic mutism. Here the patient is conscious, with eyes open, but displays a paucity of movement, incontinence and a profound indifference to the external world with an absence of spontaneous speech, and an inability to attend to such basic functions as eating, drinking and continence.

Frontal tests: an anatomical taxonomy

A fundamental neuroanatomical distinction can be made between the dorsolateral prefrontal cortex (DLPFC) and the ventral prefrontal cortex (VPFC). These two areas are also functionally differentiated. Thus the DLPFC is associated with spatial and conceptual reasoning processes while the VPFC, by virtue of its origin in the paleocortex and rich connections with limbic structures, is central to emotional control and behavior regulation, including stimulus reward associations (Rolls, 2000). While experimental research in the neurosciences has been successful in teasing out these frontal demarcations, this has not always translated into clinically meaningful and accessible tests suited to the bedside or consulting room, particularly in relation to VPFC function (Stuss and Levine, 2002). This translational limitation also applies to one additional frontal subdivision. Cognitive scientists regard the most anterior, teleological aspects of the VPFC, termed the frontal poles, as uniquely involved in self-awareness and autonoetic ('self knowing') consciousness (Tulving, 1985).

A description of the various experimental paradigms that define these frontal subdivisions has been articulated by Stuss and Levine (2002). In describing these tests and the deficits elicited, it is important to remember that lesions frequently encroach on more than one anatomical area, thereby obfuscating the presentation. Cognizant of this, three main cognitive tasks have been linked to the dorsolateral prefrontal cortex, namely language functions, memory (including working memory) and certain aspects of attention.

Dorsolateral prefrontal cortex
Language

Grossly abnormal aspects of language, for example the non-fluent aphasia of Broca, will not be addressed here, as the contributing pathology lies outside the DLPFC. One aspect of language that is, however, affected by DLPFC pathology is verbal fluency, which can be readily assessed by a test of phonological or letter fluency. A widely used and easily applied cognitive test that challenges many of these functions is the Controlled Oral Word Association Test (COWAT) (Benton, 1968), also known as the Letter Fluency Test or FAS-Test. Here the subject is required to produce orally as many words as possible beginning with the letters F, A and S. These letters are the most commonly used, although Benton et al (1983) have used C, F, L and P, R, W. With the patient seated the following instructions are given by the examiner with a stop-watch at the ready: *'I will say a letter of the alphabet. Then I want you to give me as many words that begin with that letter as quickly as you can. For instance, if I say "B", you might give me "bad, battle, bed ..." I do not want you to use words that are proper names such as "Boston, Bob or Buick". Also, do not use the same word again with a different ending such as "eat" and "eating". Any questions? (Pause) Begin when I say the letter. The first letter is F. Go ahead'.* Begin timing immediately. Allow 1 minute for each letter (F, A and S). Say 'Fine' or 'Good' after each 1-minute performance. If patients discontinue before the end of the minute, they should be encouraged to persevere with the task. If silence ensues for more than 15 seconds, repeat the basic instructions. The examiner must either write down the patient's responses, or, if they are too quick, mark a series of checks per word. At the end of the 3 minutes, the numbers of words are added together and the presence of perseverative responses (i.e. repetition of the same word) noted. There are published normative data, age-corrected, with which to compare the results.

The COWAT is considered a sensitive index of brain dysfunction (Crockett et al, 1990; Mutchnick et al, 1991) and there are a number of studies demonstrating an association between frontal pathology and impaired performance on the COWAT. There is, however, disagreement about whether frontal laterality is important. Studies have found abnormal performance on the COWAT irrespective of side of frontal lesion (Bruyer and Tuyumbu, 1980; Miceli et al, 1981), while others have noted an association with either left-sided or bilateral lesions (Benton, 1968; Parks et al, 1988; Perret, 1974; Ramier and Hecaen, 1970, Ruff et al, 1994). A more specific link between poor performance on the COWAT and inferomedial frontal pathology has been reported (Crowe, 1992). The results of these studies showing a predilection for frontal pathology have been offset by others suggesting a more widespread cerebral involvement. In a wide-ranging investigation of brain correlates of cognitive abnormalities in multiple sclerosis, poor verbal fluency correlated with atrophy affecting the anterior corpus callosum (Pozzilli et al, 1991). Temporal lobe involvement with impaired COWAT performance has also been reported (Pachana et al, 1996).

Imaging activation studies in healthy controls also reflect these divergent findings with performance linked to the dorsolateral prefrontal cortex (Cantor-Graae et al, 1993; Warkentin et al, 1991) and bilateral frontal and temporal areas (Parks et al, 1988).

These seemingly discrepant findings become easier to comprehend when viewed alongside the anatomy of the dorsolateral prefrontal circuit, incorporating as it does frontal and subcortical structures with their direct and indirect connections to the hypothalamus and medial temporal lobes (hippocampus). Thus, a lesion situated at any point along this richly interconnected pathway may lead to difficulties in generating lists of words. An example is Huntington's disease where a primary striatal abnormality, i.e. the involvement of the caudate nucleus, may produce impaired verbal fluency and a dysexecutive syndrome considered typical of frontal deficits.

Memory

Pathology localized to the frontal lobes does not produce amnesia per se. Rather, the importance of the frontal lobes in memory function is one of control (Moscovitch and Winocur, 1992). There is a plethora of experimental memory paradigms that probe amnesia or deficits in associative learning, an aspect of cognition more closely allied with medial temporal lobe functioning. These tests do not generally shed light on the strategic process explaining how memory operates. Neuropsychological tests, such as the California Verbal Learning Test (CVLT) (Delis et al, 1987) and the use of activation functional brain imaging studies have, however, confirmed the importance of the DLPFC in encoding, retrieval and, to a lesser extent, recognition aspects of memory (Stuss and Levine, 2002). There are also empirical data highlighting laterality effects, with the right prefrontal cortex strongly associated with episodic memory retrieval (Tulving et al, 1994).

The role of the DLPFC in working memory is not, however, as clear. Working memory, which may be roughly defined as that aspect of memory held 'on line', is subject to frontal control but, as in other aspects of memory discussed above, the DLPFC is not concerned with storage capacity (for example a 7-digit telephone number), but rather with the control and manipulation of that memory held on line (Stuss and Levine, 2002). The Digit Span Test (Wechsler, 1987), whereby a subject is required to repeat a series of single digits spaced at 1-second intervals, taps into more posterior brain regions (viz parietal lobes). However, asking the subject to repeat the digits in the reverse order does measure the manipulation of the information stored in working memory and is thus linked to DLPFC control. Published normative data are available for the Digit Span Test. An additional method of testing how memory processing operates is to challenge a subject with a supraspan test, i.e. one that provides information exceeding the capacity of working memory. Given that the average digit span in a middle-aged adult is 7 digits forwards, providing a list of numbers in excess of this will demand additional strategies from a subject when challenged with recall.

Attention

The attention neural network is widely dispersed, which can make cerebral lateralization a hazardous task. For example, consider the network subserving spatial attention that involves the posterior parietal cortex, frontal eye fields, anterior cingulate and reticular activating system (Mesulam, 1981). The role of the frontal lobes here is similar to that in memory, namely one of control. In this way it oversees various aspects of attention that include switching, selection in the face of distractors and vigilance, i.e. sustained attention (Stuss and Levine, 2002).

There are two widely used tests that probe subjects' ability to shift the focus of their attention, namely the Wisconsin Card Sort Test (WCST) (Grant and Berg, 1948), and the Trail Making Test, part B (Reitan and Wolfson, 1985). First formulated by Berg in 1948, the WCST has subsequently been revised and expanded (Heaton, 1981). Subjects are given a pack of 128 cards which contain four symbols, namely star, cross, triangle and circle, in four colors, namely red, blue, yellow and green. Four stimulus cards are placed before them in the following left-to-right order: one red triangle, two green stars, three yellow crosses and four blue circles. Subjects are then instructed to match each consecutive card from the deck with one of the four stimulus cards, in whichever way they think they match. Subjects are told whether they are right or wrong and the correct sorting principle is never revealed. Once a certain number of correct responses are made to the initial sorting principle, the sorting principle is changed, e.g. from color to form. This occurs without warning and subjects have only the examiner's responses to alert them of the change. The test proceeds in similar fashion through a series of shifts in set, namely color, form, number, etc. The test provides scores on such indices as the number of categories completed, the total number of errors made and the number of perseverative responses made, to name but three of the most sensitive indices of conceptual reasoning.

Performance on the WCST has been linked to the functional integrity of the DLPFC (Heaton et al, 1993), although there are dissenting voices (Anderson et al, 1991). A positron emission tomography (PET) study that demonstrated the inability of schizophrenic patients to match the performance of healthy subjects on the WCST noted a robust association between deficits and hypoperfusion in the DLPFC (Weinberger et al, 1986), findings subsequently replicated by others (Berman et al, 1995). Evidence suggests that the DLPFC is particularly relevant in shifting set from color to form, for example (termed extra-dimensional), rather than from color to color (e.g. green to yellow, termed intra-dimensional) (Rogers et al, 2000).

A computerized version of the test is now in the public domain and comes with an automated scoring system.

A second, widely used test that taps similar cognitive attributes is the Trail Making Test, part B (Reitan and Wolfson, 1985). In part A, the subject is given a pencil and told to mark a sequential trail on a piece of paper that contains a series of consecutive numbers scattered in random fashion. Thus, the correct trail would proceed as $1 \rightarrow 2 \rightarrow 3 \rightarrow 4 \rightarrow 5$ and so on. The test is timed. In Trail Making B, a consecutive series of numbers and letters are scattered on the page and the subject is now instructed to proceed in a sequence that alternates numbers with letters $1 \rightarrow A \rightarrow 2 \rightarrow B \rightarrow 3 \rightarrow C \rightarrow 4 \rightarrow D \rightarrow 5 \rightarrow E$ and so on. Once again the test is timed, unlike the WCST. Evidence suggests that failure to switch set in part B and the inability to sustain attention over the duration of the study is associated with DLPFC dysfunction (Stuss et al, 2001).

One of the drawbacks to this test is that speed of performance is dependent on good motor co-ordination which creates problems in patients with neuropsychiatric disorders such as multiple sclerosis and Parkinson's disease. However, Trail Making A may be regarded as a control task for time and therefore used to factor out this potential confounder (Stuss et al, 2001).

Selective attention may be assessed with the Stroop Test (Stroop, 1935). It assesses the ability to focus attention on one attribute of a compound stimulus (the color in which words are written) and simultaneously to ignore another competing attribute (the meaning of the word).

The effect is produced by the primacy, in information processing terms, of semantic content over physical features. Poor performance is indicated by either slow speed, frequent errors or both. In a computerized version of the test used in our research laboratory subjects are first asked to read a list of words denoting a series of colors. This first control paradigm provides an estimate of reading speed. In the second control paradigm they are asked to name the color of each square in a series of colored squares. In the third task, the actual Stroop paradigm, subjects are presented with the names of colors written in different colors. What they have to do is say the color the word is written in, not the color named by the word. Thus, although the first word in Figure 5.1 says red, the correct answer is yellow.

Results from experimental psychology have implicated two frontal areas in the performance of the Stroop test, namely the DLPFC (right or left) and the anterior cingulate cortex (Bench et al, 1993; Stuss et al, 1981; Vendrell et al, 1995). While patients with frontal damage are slow on all three parts of the test, the DLPFC appears to be linked to speed of

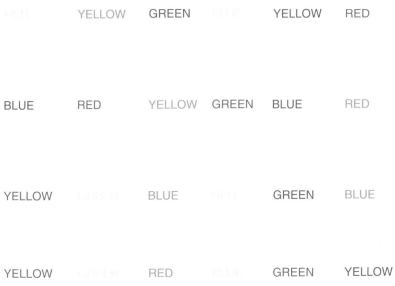

Figure 5.1 *The Stroop Test. Subjects have to give the color the word is written in and not the name as written.*

color-naming (paradigms 1 and 2), whereas the superior medial areas control selective attention (paradigm 3).

Attention sustained over time is termed vigilance (Strub and Black, 1977) and appears mediated by frontal regions, particularly the right DLPFC (Stuss and Levine, 2002). Right frontal activation is enhanced under two conditions: when the target complexity is increased, as in a choice- versus simple-reaction-time test (Reuckert and Grafman, 1996) and when the speed of the stimulus is reduced, i.e. slow, sustained tasks instead of rapidly paced ones (Reuckert and Grafman, 1998).

The ventral prefrontal cortex

In contrast to the DLPFC, the ventral prefontal cortex controls emotions, self-regulation and decision-making processes. Psychometrically testing the functional integrity of these personal attributes is almost exclusively within the research domain.

Decision-making can be tested using the 'Gambling Task', a novel paradigm that challenges real-life decision-making (Bechara et al, 1994). This test has now been computerized to facilitate presentation and takes approximately 15–20 minutes to complete. Subjects are given $200 of 'virtual' money before testing begins and instructed to select from four identical decks of cards with the simple instruction to maximize gains and minimize losses. Each deck has a programmed system of differing monetary awards and penalties. However, the subject does not know what the program is in advance and has to work out, as the test progresses, which decks are advantageous or punitive. The final score, after 100 cards are chosen, is the difference between cards drawn from the 'good' and 'bad' decks.

Behavioral self-regulation is also allied to VPFC function. Stuss and Levine (2002) have coined the term 'self-regulatory disorder' (SRD) describing an 'inability to regulate behavior according to internal goals and restraints'. The process of self-regulation goes awry when subjects fail to maintain consistent self-representations and use this self-information to inform their own decision-making in the appropriateness of their social responses. Such behavior is most noticeable in unstructured social situations where an impulsivity often overwhelms the decision-making process, with adverse long-term consequences. Conversely, highly structured situations induce restraint in patients with SRD. This is turn may superficially obscure their often catastrophic social deficits (Mesulam, 1986). Self-regulatory behavior cannot be tested clinically. While a laboratory measure has been developed, termed the Strategy Application Test (Levine et al, 1998), a detailed history from a close informant of the patient provides the necessary clues to diagnosis.

A straightforward means of challenging orbitofrontal functional integrity is to test olfaction. One detailed assessment is the University of Pennsylvania Smell Identification Test (UPSIT) (Doty, 1983; Doty et al, 1984). This scratch and sniff test contains 40 odors, some common and others rare. After sniffing an odor, the subject is presented with a choice of four possible answers that are read aloud. Each odor is presented unilaterally, 20 per nostril. Evidence points towards the importance of the medial orbitofrontal areas in mediating olfaction (Jones-Gotman and Zatorre, 1988; Zatorre and Jones-Gotman, 1991).

The cognitive relevance of a further frontal subdivision, namely the frontal poles, has been emphasized. This region is considered important in memory of self, termed episodic memory. Once again, a laterality effect has been described, with the right frontal pole associated with recall of biographical information (Craik et al, 1999). Autonoetic knowledge, the process of knowing self, is also intricately embedded in right polar function (Tulving, 1985). A method for assessing episodic memory that consists of a detailed autobiographical questionnaire is recommended for patients with non-dominant prefrontal pathology (Kopelman et al, 1989). Finally, this same anatomical region is important in determining a subject's ability to appreciate humor (Shammi and Stuss, 1999).

In summary, the following tests have been provided as indicators of frontal function: the Controlled Oral Word Association Test (COWAT); Digit Span reversed; supraspan tasks; the Wisconsin Card Sort Test; the Trail Making Test, part B; the Stroop Test; Choice Reaction Time tests; the Gambling Task; the Smell Test; the Strategy Application Test; and the Autobiographical Questionnaire. Of these, only three (COWAT, Digit Span reversed, Autobiographical Questionnaire) are readily presentable at the bedside, with the remainder being used in research settings. A further delimiter is the recognition that these tests tap into multiple cognitive domains and therefore involve brain regions beyond the frontal lobes. A useful rule of thumb, cognitively speaking, is that the more complex the task, the more likely it is to involve frontal regions (Stuss and Levine, 2002). This in itself does not, however, guarantee regional specificity. While they are of inestimable significance in helping to unravel the mysteries of cognitive neuroscience, the esoteric nature of most of these tests places their utility beyond the reach of clinicians. For this reason, a more strictly translational research effort has been devoted to the establishment of relatively brief, doable, bedside-friendly tests of frontally mediated cognitive abilities.

Frontal lobe clinical batteries

A multicenter attempt at developing a bedside mental state assessment of frontal lobe involvement focused on a methodology that emphasized brevity and an absence of materials and equipment (Ettlin et al, 2000). Four groups of subjects were examined: those with frontal (n = 27), non-frontal (n = 25) and mixed, frontal and non-frontal (n = 17) lesions plus a group of healthy controls (n = 48). Patients with aphasia, an age over 70 years, dementia, psychiatric disease and substance abuse were excluded. A detailed literature review of putative frontal lobe tasks led to the selection of 22 tests, which were then combined with 12 items from the Neurobehavioral Rating Scale (NRS) (Levin et al, 1987) and seven dysfunctional aspects of spontaneous speech and narrative discourse. To score the NRS the patients' own observations were supplemented by those of their relatives, nurses, physicians and the examiner's evaluations during testing. Given that the aim was the production of a battery that had the highest sensitivity and specificity for detecting frontal lobe pathology, those test items that best discriminated between frontal and non-frontal lesions were chosen.

The final result was a compendium of 14 tests, incorporating 56 variables. The clinical utility of these measures was enhanced by the development of a simple scoring system. The tests include the items in Table 5.1.

Table 5.1 Frontal lobe clinical battery of tests. (Reproduced from Eltlin et al, 2000, with permission from Arnold Publishers.)

	Pathological range	*Score value*
Serial sevens		
Errors	> 2	1
Time (s)	> 88	1
Error pattern	all	1
Reverse spelling		
Errors	> 1	1
Time (s)	> 6	1
Not completed		1
Weekdays in reverse		
Errors	> 0	1
Time (s)	> 7	1
Months in reverse		
Errors	> 1	1
Time (s)	> 24	1
Error pattern	all	1
Trail Making Test A		
Errors	> 0	1
Time (s)	> 23	1
Error pattern	all	1
Trail Making Test B		
Errors	> 1	1
Time (s)	> 106	1
Error pattern	all	1
Grasp Reflex		
Right hand	present	1
Left hand	present	1
Rhythm tapping		
Not completed		1
Error pattern	all	2

Table 5.1 Continued

	Pathological range	Score value
Luria's hand sequences 2-step		
Fluency	decreased	2
Luria's hand sequences 3-step		
Trials right hand	> 3	1
Not completed		2
Trials left hand	> 2	1
Not completed		2
Fluency	decreased	1
Error pattern		
Go–no go		
Errors	> 1	1
Error pattern	all	1
Alternating pattern		
Errors	all	1
Five-point test		
Correct	< 7	1
Word list learning		
Correct, trial 1	< 4	1
Correct, trial 2	< 6	1
Correct, trial 3	< 7	1
Correct, trial 4	< 8	1
Correct, recall	< 6	1
Neurobehavioral Rating Scale		
Emotional withdrawal	present	2
Depressive mood	present	2
Decreased initiative	present	2
Motor retardation	present	2
Blunted affect	present	2
Lability of mood	present	2
Disinhibition	present	2

Table 5.1 Continued

	Pathological range	Score value
Hostility/uncooperativeness	present	2
Excitement	present	2
Inattention	present	2
Poor planning	present	2
Inaccurate insight	present	2
Spontaneous speech		
Reduced production	present	1
Fixation on details	present	1
Lack of distance	present	1
Discursive discourse	present	1
Incoherence	present	1
Missing chronology	present	1
Perseveration	present	1

A total frontal lobe score (FLS) of ≥ 12 indicates frontal lobe damage.

The frontal lobe score (FLS) has a sensitivity of 77.7% in detecting frontal lesions, i.e. it correctly identified 21 out of 27 patients with well-demarcated frontal lesions. When the mixed group was added to this group, the sensitivity was reduced slightly to 71.1%. The specificity was 84%. In healthy controls the specificity was 100% (none had frontal pathology). The results indicate that the ability to detect frontal dysfunction is enhanced when cognitive measures are supplemented with behavioral and language indices.

While the sensitivity and specificity of the FLS are respectable, almost one in four patients with frontal lesions is missed, raising the question to what degree the scale compares with the more complex psychometric tests outlined earlier in this chapter. In answer to this query, the authors undertook a subsequent validation study comparing the sensitivity of the FLS to the Wisconsin Card Sort and Stroop tests (Wildgruber et al, 2000). A sample of 108 subjects (26 with frontal lesions, 28 with non-frontal cerebral lesions, 31 with mixed frontal and non-frontal lesions,

Table 5.2 Evaluation of frontal lobe score (FLS), Wisconsin Card Sort Test (WCST) and Stroop test.

	Frontal lesions only	*Frontal lesions vs healthy controls*	*Frontal lesions vs non-frontal lesions*
FLS	Sensitivity 92.3%	Specificity 100%	Specificity 75.0%
WCST	Sensitivity 65.4%	Specificity 60.9%	Specificity 53.6%
Stroop	Sensitivity 30.8%	Specificity 95.7%	Specificity 92.9%

and 23 healthy controls) completed the FLS, WCST and Stroop test. The results of the three tests are summarized in Table 5.2.

The conclusion reached was that the FLS was superior to both the WCST and Stroop test in screening for frontal lesions. Notwithstanding this impressive validation, the 22% false-negative rate speaks to the importance of adjunct investigations such as computed tomography and magnetic resonance imaging brain scans in arriving at a more complete assessment.

Other, less comprehensive, 'frontal' batteries have been developed and warrant consideration. The Frontal Assessment Battery (FAB) is a six-item, bedside test that takes no longer than 10 minutes to complete (Dubois et al, 2000). The tests challenge conceptualization, mental flexibility, motor programming, inhibitory control and environmental autonomy, considered prototypical frontal functions. The six tests are as follows:

1. *Similarities (conceptualization)*
   In what way are the following alike?
      A banana and an orange
      A table and a chair
      A tulip, rose and daisy
   Score: three correct = 3; two correct = 2; one correct = 1; none correct = 0.
2. *Lexical fluency (mental flexibility)*
   The number of words beginning with the letter S in 1 minute (excluding surnames and proper nouns)
   Score: > 9 words = 3; 6–9 words = 2; 3–5 words = 1; < 3 words = 0.

3. *Motor series (programming)*

   Luria's three-step procedure (fist, edge, palm)

   Score: six consecutive series alone = 3; at least three consecutive series alone = 2; fails alone, but performs three consecutive series with the examiner = 1; cannot perform with examiner = 0.

4. *Conflicting instructions (sensitivity to interference)*

   'Tap twice when I tap once' alternating with 'tap once when I tap twice'.

   The following sequence of taps is given 1–1–2–1–2–2–2–1–1–2

   Score: no error = 3; 1–2 errors = 2; > 2 errors = 1; subject taps like examiner four consecutive times = 0.

5. *Go–no go (inhibitory control)*

   'Tap once when I tap once' interspersed with 'Do not tap when I tap twice'.

   The following sequence of taps is given: 1–1–2–1–2–2–2–1–1–2

   Score: no error = 3; 1–2 errors = 2; > 2 errors – 1, subject taps like examiner four consecutive times = 0.

6. *Prehension behavior (environmental autonomy)*

   The examiner sits before the patient who sits with palms up on his/her knees. The examiner then brings his/her hands close to those of the patient and touches the palms to see how the patient will respond spontaneously. If the earlier instruction not to take the examiner's hands is ignored, repeat the test with the instruction 'Now, do not take my hands'.

   Score: does not take hands = 3; patient hesitates and asks what he/she has to do = 2; patient takes the hands without hesitation=1; patient takes the examiner's hands even when instructed not to do so = 0.

The FAB was validated (Dubois et al, 2000) in a sample of 42 healthy control subjects and 121 patients with Parkinson's disease (n = 24), multi-system atrophy (n = 6), corticobasilar degeneration (n = 21), progressive supranuclear palsy (n = 47) and frontotemporal dementia (n = 23). Other cognitive measures included the Mini Mental State Examination (MMSE) (Folstein et al, 1975) and the Mattis Dementia Rating Scale (DRS) (Mattis, 1988). Good correlations were reported between the FAB and the DRS ($r = 0.82$; $p < 0.01$), the number of criteria ($r = 0.77$; $p < 0.01$) and perseverative errors on the WCST ($r = 0.68$; $p < 0.01$). When it came to predictors of frontal involvement, these variables accounted for 79% of the variance with age and the MMSE having no effect. The absence of an association between the FAB and the MMSE, the latter an indicator of more global cognitive dysfunction, indicates the relative sensitivity of the FAB to frontal dysfunction.

The aim of this chapter is not to provide a review of all the many frontal batteries published, but rather to highlight a few of those with impressive sensitivity/specificity ratios that are readily presentable at the bedside. While there is broad consensus on what the processes are that underlie frontally mediated cognitive function, the choice of tests varies according to the preferences of the clinicians or researchers. Indeed, some approaches focus exclusively on behavioral measures, arguing that the most prominent early signs of frontal lobe involvement are behavioral, not cognitive, with alterations in personality alerting family members to the impending problem. One such scale is the Frontal Behavioral Inventory (FBI) (Kertesz et al, 1997). Drawing on their clinical observations and published research data defining the phenomenology of frontal psychopathology, the authors divide behaviors into what they term deficit and positive subgroups. Each group comprises 12 sometimes-overlapping behaviors. For the positive group, these include perseveration, irritability, excessive or childish jocularity, irresponsibility, inappropriateness, impulsivity, restlessness, aggression, hyperorality, hypersexuality, utilization behavior and incontinence. The deficit group comprises apathy, aspontaneity, indifference, inflexibility, concreteness, personal neglect, disorganization, inattention, loss of insight, logopenia, verbal apraxia and alien hand. Behavior is scored on a four-point Likert scale (none, mild, moderate or severe) and a cut-off score of 30 is used to signify predominantly frontal type behaviors.

In a later study (Kertesz et al, 2000) the Frontal Behavioral Inventory was given to the caregivers of 108 patients with the following disorders: frontotemporal dementia (FTD) (n = 26), vascular dementia (n = 16), Alzheimer's disease (n = 38), primary progressive aphasia (n = 11) and depressive illness (n = 17). The scale differentiated patients with FTD from all other conditions with varying degrees of success, none of which fell below a significance value of 0.001. Thus, the percentages of patients classified correctly with FTD versus another disorder were as follows: vascular dementia, 85.7%; Alzheimer's dementia, 100%; primary progressive aphasia, 100%; depressive illness, 90.7%. Only with respect to vascular dementia did the false-positive rate of 19% challenge the scale's specificity. It is, however, possible that the one-in-five misdiagnosis rate may reflect vascular pathology encroaching on the frontal lobes, rather than any construct weakness in the scale. Nevertheless, some signs were more powerful indices of frontal involvement than others, with perseveration, indifference, inattention, inappropriateness and lack of insight particularly pertinent to frontally mediated behavioral aberration. The breakdown in insight emphasizes the importance of access to an informant, something equally relevant to measures such as the Neurobehavioral Rating Scale, part of the FLS described earlier. For those readers wishing to use the FBI, the text for the questions is within the public domain (Kertesz et al, 1997).

Conclusions

In this chapter we have reviewed the psychometric and behavioral data pertaining to frontal lobe function. The complexity of mentation ensures that there is no single measure that is pathognomonic of frontal disease. Nevertheless, various combinations of paradigms (many of them readily presentable at the bedside) and informant-based behavioral questionnaires have been used to create an index of frontal dysfunction boasting an impressive sensitivity and specificity. However, from the perspective of a clinician in search of a neurological or psychiatric diagnosis, these batteries should not be used in isolation, for they cannot be considered the final arbiter of cerebral localization. They are but one means, albeit an important one, in helping to make sense of a particular neurobehavioral presentation. These inventories should therefore be one part of a patient work-up that includes a thorough history, neurological examination, mental state assessment and, wherever possible, neuroimaging.

References

Anderson SW, Damasio H, Jones RD, Tranel D (1991) Wisconsin Card Sorting Test performance as a measure of frontal lobe damage. *J Clin Exp Neuropsychol* **13**:909–922.

Bechara A, Damasio AR, Damasio H, Anderson SW (1994) Insensitivity to future consequences following damage to human prefrontal cortex. *Cognition* **50**:7–15.

Bench CJ, Frith CD, Grasby PM, Friston KJ, Paulesu E et al (1993) Investigations of the functional anatomy of attention using the Stroop test. *Neuropsychologia* **31**:907–922.

Benton AL (1968) Differential behavioral effects in frontal lobe disease. *Neuropsychologia* **6**:53–60.

Benton AL, Hamsher K, Sivan AB (1983) *Multilingual Aphasia Examination*. Iowa City, IA: AJA Associates.

Berg EA (1948) A simple objective technique for measuring flexibility in thinking. *J Gen Psychol* **39**:15–22.

Berman KF, Ostrem JL, Randolph C, Gold J, Goldberg TE et al (1995) Physiological activation of a cortical network during performance of the Wisconsin Card Sorting Test: a positron emission tomography study. *Neuropsychologia* **33**:1027–1046.

Bruyer R, Tuyumbu B (1980) Fluence verbale et lesions du cortex cerebrale: performances et types d'erreurs. *Encephale* **6**:287–297.

Cantor-Graae E, Warkentin S, Franzen G, Risberg J (1993) Frontal lobe challenge: A comparison of activation procedures during rCBF measurement in normal subjects. *Neuropsychiatry Neuropsychol Behav Neurol* **6**:83–92.

Craik FIM, Moroz TM, Moscovitch M, Stuss DT, Winocur G et al (1999) In search of the self: a positron emission tomography study. *J Psychol Sci* **10**:27–35.

Crockett DJ, Hurwitz T, Vernon-Wilkinson R (1990) Differences in neuropsychological performance in psychiatric, anterior- and posterior-cerebral dysfunctioning groups. *Int J Neurosci* **52**:45–57.

Crowe SF (1992) Dissociation of two frontal lobe syndromes by a test of verbal fluency. *J Clin Exp Neuropsychol* **14**:327–339.

Delis DC, Kramer JH, Kaplan E, Ober BA (1987) *California Verbal Learning Test: Adult Version Manual*. San Antonio, TX: The Psychological Corporation.

Doty RL (1983) *The University of Pennsylvania Smell Identification Test Administration Manual*. Philadelphia: Sensonics.

Doty RL, Shaman P, Dann M (1984) Development of the University of Pennsylvania Smell Identification Test: a standardized microencapsulated test of olfactory function. *Physiol Behav* **32**:489–502.

Dubois B, Slachevsky A, Litvan I, Pillon B (2000) The FAB: A frontal assessment battery at bedside. *Neurology* **55**:1621–1626.

Ettlin TM, Kischka U, Beckson M, Gaggiotti M, Rauchfleisch U et al (2000) The Frontal Lobe Score: part I: construction of a mental status of frontal systems. *Clin Rehabil* **14**:260–271.

Folstein MF, Folstein SE, McHugh PR (1975) 'Mini-mental state'. A practical method for grading the cognitive state of patients for the clinician. *J Psychiatr Res* **12**:189–198.

Grant DA, Berg EA (1984) A behavioral analysis of degree of impairment and ease of shifting to new responses in a Weigl-type card sorting problem. *J Exp Psychol* **39**:404–411.

Heaton RK (1981) *Wisconsin Card Sorting Test Manual*. Odessa, FL: Psychological Assessment Resources.

Heaton RK Chelune GJ, Talley JL, Kay GG, Curtis G (1993) *Wisconsin Card Sorting Test (WCST) Manual Revised and Expanded*. Odessa, FL: Psychological Assessment Resources.

Jones-Gotman M, Zatorre RJ (1988) Olfactory identification deficits in patients with focal cerebral excision. *Neuropsychologia* **26**:387–400.

Kertesz A, Davidson W, Fox H (1997) Frontal behavioral inventory: Diagnostic criteria for frontal lobe dementia. *Can J Neurol Sci* **24**:29–36.

Kertesz A, Nadkarni N, Davidson W, Thomas AW (2000) The Frontal Behavioral Inventory in the differential diagnosis of frontotemporal dementia. *J Int Neuropsychol Soc* **6**:460–468.

Kopelman MD, Wilson BA, Baddeley AD (1989) The autobiographical memory interview: a new assessment of autobiographical and personal semantic memory in amnesic patients. *J Clin Exp Neuropsychol* **11**:724–744.

Levin HS, High WM, Goethe KE, Sisson RA, Overall JE et al (1987) The neuro-behavioral rating scale: assessment of the behavioral sequelae of head injury by the clinician. *J Neurol Neurosurg Psychiatry* **50**:183–193.

Levine B, Stuss DT, Milberg WP, Alexander MP, Schwartz M et al (1998) The effects of focal and diffuse brain damage on strategy application: evidence from focal lesions, traumatic brain injury, and normal aging. *J Int Neuropsychol Soc* **4**:247–264.

Malloy PF, Richardson ED (1994) Assessment of frontal lobe functions. *J Neuropsychiatry Clin Neurosci* **6**:399–410.

Mattis S (1988) *Dementia Rating Scale*. Odessa, FL: Psychological Assessment Resources.

Mesulam M-M (1981) A cortical network for directed attention and unilateral neglect. *Ann Neurol* **10**:309–325.

Mesulam M-M (1986) Frontal cortex and behavior. *Ann Neurol* **19**:320–325.

Miceli G, Caltagirone C, Gainotti G, Masullo C, Silveri MC (1981) Neuropsychological correlates of localized cerebral lesions in non-aphasic brain-damaged patients. *J Clin Neuropsychol* **3**:53–63.

Moscovitch M, Winocur G (1992) The neuropsychology of memory and aging. In Salthouse TA, Craik FIM (eds) *The Handbook of Aging and Cognition*. Hillsdale, NJ: Erlbaum, 1992: 315–372.

Mutchnick MG, Ross LK, Long CJ (1991) Decision strategies for cerebral dysfunction IV: Determination of cerebral dysfunction. *Arch Clin Neuropsychol* **6**:259–270.

Pachana NA, Boone KB, Miller BL, Cummings JL, Berman N (1996) Comparison of neuropsychological functioning in Alzheimer's disease and frontotemporal dementia. *J Int Neuropsychol Soc* **2**:505–510.

Parks RW, Loewenstein DA, Dodrill KL, Barker WW, Yoshii F et al (1988) Cerebral metabolic effects of a verbal fluency test: A PET scan study. *J Clin Exp Neuropsychol* **10**:565–575.

Perret E (1974) The left frontal lobe of man and the suppression of habitual responses in verbal categorical behavior. *Neuropsychologia* **12**:323–330.

Pozzilli C, Batianello S, Padovani A, Passifiume D (1991) Anterior corpus callosum atrophy and verbal fluency in multiple sclerosis. *Cortex* **27**:441–445.

Ramier A-M, Hecaen H (1970) Role respectif des attaintes frontales et la lateralisation lésionelle dans les deficits de la 'fluence verbale'. *Rev Neurol (Paris)* **123**:17–22.

Reitan RM, Wolfson D (1985) *The Halstead-Reitan Neuropsychological Test Battery.* Tucson, AZ: Neuropsychology Press, 61–64.

Reuckert L, Grafman J (1996) Sustained attention deficits in patients with right frontal lesions. *Neuropsychologia* **34**:953–963.

Reuckert L, Grafman J (1998) Sustained attention deficits in patients with lesions of posterior cortex. *Neuropsychologia* **36**:653–660

Rogers RD, Andrews TC, Grasby PM, Brooks DJ, Robbins TW (2000) Contrasting cortical and subcortical activations produced by attentional-set shifting and reversal learning in humans. *J Cogn Neurosci* **12**:142–162.

Rolls ET (2000) The orbitofrontal cortex and reward. *Cereb Cortex* **10**:284–294.

Ruff RM, Allen CC, Farrow CE, Niemann H, Wylie T (1994) Figural fluency: Differential impairment in patients with left versus right frontal lobe lesions. *Arch Clin Neuropsychol* **9**:41–55.

Shammi P, Stuss DT (1999) Humour appreciation: a role of the right frontal lobe. *Brain* **122**:657–666.

Stroop JR (1935) Studies of interference in serial verbal reaction. *J Exp Psychol* **18**:643–662.

Strub RL, Black FW (1977) *The Mental Status Examination in Neurology.* Philadelphia: FA Davis.

Stuss DT, Levine B (2002) Adult clinical neuropsychology: Lessons from studies of the frontal lobes. *Annu Rev Psychol* **53**:401–433.

Stuss DT, Benson DF, Kapan EF, Weir WS, Della Malva C (1981) Leucotomized and nonleucotomized schizophrenics: comparison on tests of attention. *Biol Psychiatry* **16**:1085–1100.

Stuss DT, Bisschop SM, Alexander MP, Levine B, Katz D et al (2001) The Trail Making Test: a study in focal lesion patients. *Psychol Assess* **13**:230–239.

Tulving E (1985) Memory and consciousness. *Can J Psychol* **26**:1–12.

Tulving E, Kapur S, Craik FIM, Moscovitch M, Houle S (1994) Hemispheric encoding/retrieval asymmetry in episodic memory: positron emission tomography findings. *Proc Natl Acad Sci USA* **91**:2016–2020.

Vendrell P, Junque C, Pujol J, Jurado MA, Molet J et al (1995) The role of prefrontal regions in the Stroop task. *Neuropsychologia* **33**:341–352.

Warkentin S, Risberg J, Nilsson A, Karlson S, Graae E (1991) Cortical activity during speech production: A study of regional cerebral blood flow in normal subjects performing a word fluency task. *Neuropsychiatry Neuropsychol Behav Neurol* **4**:305–316.

Wechsler D (1987) *Wechsler Memory Scale-Revised.* San Antonio, TX: The Psychological Corporation.

Weinberger DR, Berman KF, Zec RF (1986) Physiologic dysfunction of dorsolateral prefrontal cortex in schizophrenia. I: Regional cerebral blood flow evidence. *Arch Gen Psychiatry* **43**:114–124.

Wildgruber D, Kischka U, Fassbender K, Ettlin TM (2000) The Frontal Lobe Score: part II: evaluation of its clinical validity. *Clin Rehabil* **14**:272–278.

Zatorre RJ, Jones-Gotman M (1991) Human olfactory discrimination after unilateral frontal or temporal lobectomy. *Brain* **114**:71–84.

chapter 6

Short cognitive screening tests and batteries

Abbreviated Mental Test

The Abbreviated Mental Test (AMT) has achieved its widest use in Great Britain and Europe but is seldom used in North America. This 10-item mental test was developed by Hodkinson (1972) and in turn was based on the instrument developed by Blessed et al (1968). In a multi-center study of mental disorders in elderly hospital inpatients under the auspices of the Royal College of Physicians, London, the original instrument consisted of 26 items. However, it was determined that the test could be reduced to 10 items and still maintain its discriminating functions (Appendices 6.1 and 6.2). The optimal cut-off for 'significant' cognitive impairment was considered to be 7/8, as this maximizes sensitivity and specificity.

The AMT has been assessed in a wide range of settings including long-stay care residential homes, general community samples and psycho-geriatric day hospital attenders (Jitapunkul et al, 1991). Consecutive patients admitted to the acute geriatric wards of the Royal London Hospital were assessed. Figure 6.1 shows the frequency of impaired cognitive functioning according to the AMT score. Table 6.1 shows the sensitivity and specificity of each item in identifying cognitive impairment, and Table 6.2 shows the domains of each of the items on the AMT including the seven-item AMT, which proved to have equivalent psychometric properties.

A survey conducted by Jitapunkul et al (1991) revealed that 80% of junior doctors did not use the test accurately. Twenty per cent of the

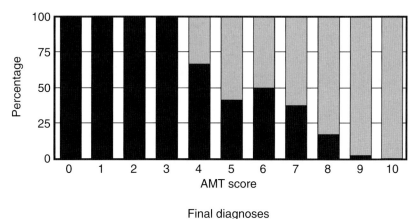

Figure 6.1 *Frequency of impaired cognitive function according to the Abbreviated Mental Test (AMT) score. (Reproduced from Jitapunkul et al, 1991, with permission from Oxford University Press.)*

Table 6.1 Sensitivity and specificity of each item on the Abbreviated Mental Test (AMT) (from Jitapunkul et al, 1991, with permission from Oxford University Press).

AMT item	Sensitivity	Specificity
1. Age	55	94
2. Time	64	87
3. Address to recall	90	54
4. Year	74	75
5. Hospital	67	88
6. Persons	53	98
7. Date of birth	52	98
8. Year of First World War	72	75
9. Monarch	72	82
10. Count 20 to 1	76	86

doctors surveyed did not know the cut-off point for abnormality and indeed a wide range of cut-off points were used by these doctors. In the study approximately 20% of cognitively normal patients were misclassified, while 8.6% of cognitively impaired patients were classified as

Table 6.2 The domains assessed by each item of the Abbreviated Mental Test (AMT) (from Jitapunkul et al, 1991, with permission from Oxford University Press).

	Concept
Seven-item AMT	
Time (2)	Time (orientation)
Address recall (3)	Attention and recent memory
Hospital (5)	Place (orientation)
Persons (6)	Person (orientation)
Date of birth (7)	Remote memory
Monarch (9)	General knowledge and memory
Count 20 to 1 (10)	Attention
Other items of the AMT	
Age (1)	Remote memory
Year (4)	Time (orientation)
Year of First World War (8)	Remote memory

normal. Like the Mini Mental State Examination (MMSE), the AMT had a good internal consistency with a high reliability co-efficient (Cronbach's alpha = 0.90).

In a study that compared the AMT to the Informant Questionnaire on Cognitive Decline in the Elderly (IQCODE) (Harwood et al, 1997), the IQCODE was more accurate than the AMT in screening for dementia. Furthermore, the IQCODE was usable in eight of 10 patients who were unable to complete the AMT. The authors suggested that the use of both the IQCODE and a brief cognitive screening test for dementia would be most useful in medical inpatients, as this would maximize the number of patients who could be successfully screened.

Trail Making Test and the Verbal Fluency Test

The Trail Making Test (Oswald and Roth, 1978; Reitan, 1958) and the Verbal Fluency Test (Isaacs and Kennie, 1973) are both frequently

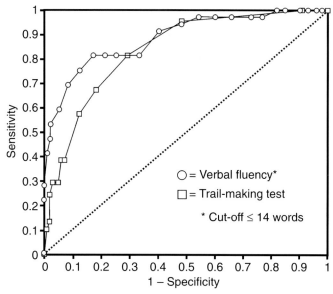

Figure 6.2 *ROC curves. (Reproduced from Heun et al, 1998, with permission from John Wiley & Sons Ltd.)*

mentioned in descriptions of effective cognitive screens (Shulman, 2000). Figure 6.2 demonstrates the receiver operating characteristic (ROC) curves for each of these tasks showing high sensitivities and specificities (Heun et al, 1998). The verbal fluency task consists of naming as many first names as possible with a particular letter and the naming of animals, each in 1 minute. This is considered an indicator of frontal lobe functioning (Isaacs and Kennie, 1973). Our experience with verbal fluency finds value in adding a phonemic prime such as any word beginning with the letter 'F' as well as a semantic prime of four-legged animals. The Trail Making Test was derived from the Reitan battery (Reitan, 1958). The best cut-off score for verbal fluency turned out to be less than 14 words per minute and corresponds to the recommendations of the original study by Isaacs and Kennie (1973). These results were similar to an earlier study by Monsch et al (1997) while Koivisto et al (1992) found comparable psychometric properties for the verbal fluency test. It has been found to correlate well with the MMSE and with a variety of clock drawing tests (Shulman, 2000).

Lorentz et al (2002) identified the following less commonly used short cognitive screens for consideration.

Short Blessed Test

The Short Blessed Test (SBT) was developed as a shorter version of the original Blessed Information Memory Concentration (BIMC) Test (Katzman et al, 1983). Six questions take approximately 5 minutes to administer and address items that include orientation (year, month, time); counting backwards from 20 to 1; months of the year backwards; and repeating a memory phrase. Correlation of the SBT with the MMSE was high ($r = 0.91$). Compared to the MMSE, the SBT was reported to be superior in detecting mild dementias and subthreshold impairment. Like the MMSE, however, it was influenced by variables of age and education.

Memory Impairment Screen

The Memory Impairment Screen (MIS) (Buschke et al, 1999) comprises four items that take approximately 4 minutes to administer. It is purported not to be affected by age or education, which is different from other cognitive screens. Compared to the three-item recall test (Kuslanski et al, 2002), it has demonstrated superior psychometric properties.

Short Test of Mental Status

The Short Test of Mental Status (STMS) is similar in its content to the MMSE including orientation, attention, learning, arithmetic, calculation, abstraction, information, construction and recall (Kokmen et al, 1991). Its sensitivity and specificity were both over 90%, using a cut-off of 29 out of a possible 38 points. However, it would appear that the results were significantly correlated with education, which is different from the Memory Impairment Screen.

Time and Change Test

Inouye et al (1998) set out to develop a performance-based indicator of cognitive functioning. They specifically chose two tasks that were deemed critical to the maintenance of independent functioning: namely telling time and the making change task.

Telling time task
A large clock-face diagram with the hands set at 11:10 is held 14 inches (35 cm) from the participant's eyes. The participant is cued: 'Please tell me what time it says on this clock'. For study purposes, the participant's response time is measured with a stopwatch that is started immediately after the cue is given. The participant is allowed two tries within a 60-second period. If the participant fails to respond correctly after two tries, the task is terminated and an error is recorded. Response time and any difficulties with the testing (e.g. vision, tremor, weakness, or pain) are also recorded.

Making change task
A standard amount of change (three quarters, seven dimes, and seven nickels) is placed on a well-lighted tabletop. The participant is cued: 'Please give me a dollar's worth of change'. For study purposes, the participant's response time is measured with a stopwatch that is started immediately after the cue is given. The participant is allowed two tries within a 180-second period. If the participant fails to respond correctly after two tries, the task is terminated and an error is recorded. As above, response time and any difficulties with the testing are also recorded.

In assessing concurrent validity, the investigators demonstrated a sensitivity of 86% and a specificity of 71% with a negative predictive value of 97%. This represents the proportion of subjects who have a negative result on the Time and Change Test and who are found not to be suffering from dementia. Of those patients who had a false-negative result, their median MMSE score was 22. Convergent validity was assessed by correlating the Time and Change Test with other cognitive measures such as the overall MMSE score (r = 0.58). The positive predictive value was only 32%, however, on this test.

As far as efficiency is concerned, time reading took 60 seconds on average and making change took 180 seconds for a total of 4 minutes for the combined tasks. The screening test was considered positive if either component was incorrect after two tries. The diagnosis of dementia was confirmed if the mean Blessed Dementia Rating Score (BDRS) was greater than 4 or if the mean BDRS was greater than 2 at the same time that an MMSE score was less than 20 and the duration of cognitive symptoms was at least 6 months.

The authors concluded that the Time and Change Test has potential value in identifying dementia in elderly hospitalized patients. Moreover, the high negative predictive value of the Time and Change Test (97%) could be useful in ruling out dementia. The Time and Change Test adds a number of additional domains compared to the MMSE, including calculation, conceptualization and visuospatial functioning. It may also prove to be useful in populations with diverse educational and cultural backgrounds, as it appears to be less influenced by educational level than the MMSE.

Brief screening batteries

The '7 Minute Screen'

The '7 Minute Screen' (7MS) (Solomon et al, 1998) purports to demonstrate a sensitivity and specificity of 100%. It also claims to be sensitive to identifying patients with mild Alzheimer's disease as defined by a MMSE score of 24 or higher. The battery consists of four brief cognitive tests: enhanced cued recall; temporal orientation; verbal fluency; and clock drawing.

Enhanced cued recall is a test that takes advantage of the finding that elderly control subjects seem to benefit from mnemonic strategies that allow storage and retrieval of information. This takes the form of reminder cues (Grober et al, 1988). *Category fluency* is the test used to incorporate word fluency, and a semantic cue of 'animals' is used in this sub-test. The *Benton Temporal Orientation Test* (Benton, 1983) reflects orientation to time by using a graduated scoring system. This is different from the MMSE orientation test, as the degree of error is scored in this sub-test. *Clock drawing* is used as a measure of visuospatial ability, but of course this test casts a wider net in terms of screening for cognitive impairment (Shulman, 2000).

The moniker '7 minute' is slightly inaccurate, in that the mean time for administration of this battery was 7 minutes and 42 seconds, actually closer to 8 minutes. The investigators obviously utilized an obscure mathematical rule for defining which minute to use.

Figure 6.3 demonstrates the frequency distributions of each of these four individual test scores for Alzheimer patients and healthy control subjects in the community.

Table 6.3 shows positive and negative predictive values for variable population base rates of dementia from 5% to 50%. The sensitivity and specificity findings are high for the full spectrum of dementia severity. The authors claim that education does not appear to influence the psychometric properties of the battery, as logistic regression analysis using education as a covariate did not affect the predictions. Similarly, adding age to the logistic regression analysis as a covariate did not alter the predictions.

It remains to be seen whether the almost 8 minutes needed for administration of this battery will result in its clinical use. Lorentz et al (2002) noted that, while age and education did not affect the psychometric properties of this test, all subjects had at least 8 years of education. Furthermore, they noted that the test requires special training and a specially designed hand-held computer which reduces its practical implementation.

The Mini-Cog

Many of the clock scoring systems are far too complicated for practical implementation or have limitations based on cultural factors and use of visual aids (Shulman, 2000). Given the limited variability of psychometric properties, no matter which scoring system has been utilized, it would make most sense to find the simplest scoring system possible.

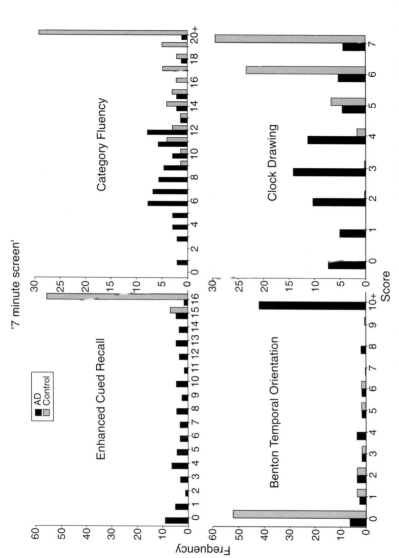

Figure 6.3 *Frequency distributions of individual test scores for patients with Alzheimer's disease (AD) and healthy control subjects. (Reproduced from Solomon et al, 1998, with permission from the American Medical Association.)*

Table 6.3 Positive and negative predictive values for variable population base rates of dementia (reproduced from Solomon et al, 1998, with permission from The American Medical Association).

Base rate	Positive predictive value (%)	Negative predictive value (%)
5	55	99
10	72	99
20	85	98
50	96	92

Borson et al (2000) have developed a very simple free-hand version of the clock drawing test. It has been validated in a diverse ethnolinguistic population and requires little language interpretation (Borson et al, 1999). In a low-education, non-English-speaking group it has proved to be superior to the MMSE in predicting dementia (Borson et al, 1999). The clock test scoring was that used by the Consortium to Establish a Registry for Alzheimer's Disease (CERAD) (Morris et al, 1989). This method of evaluation yields four possible scores based on an overall impression of the clock (0 = normal to 3 = severe impairment). The standard applied for normal rating (0) includes the requirement that numbers be present in the current sequence and position and, second, that hands readably display the specified time. In their analysis, the data were reduced to binary scores of normal (0) and abnormal (1–3). This methodology avoids the cumbersome and often ambiguous scoring systems.

In a previous study, the overall sensitivity of the CERAD scoring method for the clock drawing test was only 79% (Borson et al, 2000). In an attempt to enhance the psychometric properties of this cognitive screening method, Borson et al (2000) added a three-item memory task based on the Cognitive Abilities Screening Instrument (CASI) (Teng et al 1994) to the clock drawing test and created a composite screening instrument which they named the 'Mini-Cog' (Figure 6.4).

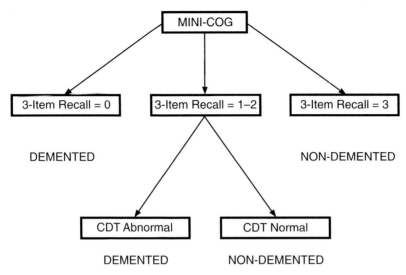

Figure 6.4 *Mini-Cog scoring algorithm. (Reproduced from Borson et al, 2000, with permission from John Wiley & Sons Ltd.)*

The relatively good psychometric properties of the clock drawing test, no matter which scoring system has been utilized, has been considered surprising in light of the fact that recent memory is not an aspect of this test (Shulman, 2000). Long considered the hallmark deficit of dementia, memory testing would seem to be critical, hence the addition of this task by Borson et al (2000). Another perspective has challenged the primacy of memory impairment in dementia, suggesting that it may be a relatively late phenomenon (Royall, 2000) (see Chapter 4).

Borson et al (2000) compared the Mini-Cog to the MMSE (Folstein et al, 1975) and to the CASI (Teng et al, 1994). The latter validated screening instrument is relatively unbiased by education even in its short form (Teng et al, 1994). Among the three screening tests, the Mini-Cog ranked first in sensitivity (99%) and diagnostic value (96%) and correctly classified subjects into those with dementia and those without dementia. While less effective in classifying non-demented subjects than the more comprehensive CASI, the Mini-Cog still had an acceptable specificity of 93%. Although the authors felt that the more significant component of the screening battery was the memory task, the clock drawing test clearly enhanced sensitivity and diagnostic value (Figure 6.4).

The Mini-Cog appears to have comparable psychometric properties to other screening instruments. However, its efficiency and practicality make it preferable, based on the preliminary data presented by Borson et al (2000). Testing time for the Mini-Cog (mean 3.2 minutes) was less than half the mean time for the MMSE (7.3 minutes) and less than one-sixth the time reported for the CASI (Teng et al, 1994). Moreover, the authors found no education or language bias. Compared to other very brief cognitive screens such as the Time and Change Test (Froehlich et al 1999), it has better sensitivity and specificity. It requires less time, equipment and training than the 7-minute screen of Solomon et al (1998).

Although it requires further replication, the Mini-Cog points in the direction of simplicity and practicality in the design of cognitive screening instruments that still maintain adequate psychometric properties. Furthermore, the results of Scanlan and Borson (2001) suggest that expert and naïve raters have high levels of concordance. The Mini-Cog has been tested only in a clinical setting and the authors suggest that, for population-based screening, the use of informants should confirm concerns about cognition prior to the initiation of the full-scale dementia work-up. Because of the diminished time involved in administering the Mini-Cog, the cost-effectiveness of this screening method will be better, assuming equal psychometric properties to more complicated and cumbersome screening tests including clock tests that require complex scoring evaluation.

The GPCOG

Similar in approach to the 'Mini-Cog', the GPCOG was designed as a brief battery for use in general practice (Brodaty et al, 2002). It includes a cognitive assessment section and an informant component that was refined to consist of nine cognitive items and six informant items (Appendix 6.3). The original battery was derived from three sources: The Cambridge Cognitive Examination (CAMCOG) (Roth et al, 1986), the Psychogeriatric Assessment Scale (Jorm et al, 1995) and the Instrumental

Activities of Daily Living (Lawton and Brody, 1969). Comparison instruments included the 10-item AMT (Hodkinson, 1972) and the MMSE (Folstein et al, 1975). DSM-IV was used as the diagnostic standard. Satisfaction questionnaires were used for both general practitioners and patients.

The refinement of the GPCOG was accomplished by the elimination of items completed by less than 5% of patients, items affirmed by less than 10% of informants or those items that did not contribute to the prediction of dementia as determined by logistic regression analysis (Brodaty et al, 2002) (Figure 6.5).

It has been argued that the GPCOG has an advantage because it combines both patient and informant data and has been validated in a primary care setting with sound psychometric properties, including sensitivity and specificity of approximately 0.85 each (Brodaty et al, 2002). The authors argue that the two-stage procedure is time efficient in that less than half of the cases required the informant to be contacted. It had

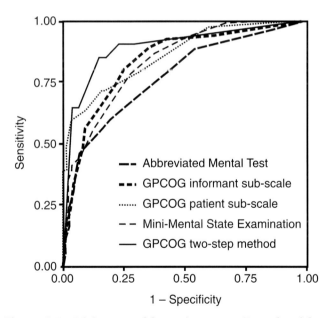

Figure 6.5 ROC curves of dementia screens. (Reproduced from Brodaty et al, 2002, with permission from Blackwell Science.)

a negative predictive value of 0.933, meaning that only 7% of patients who were identified as non-demented by the GPCOG actually did suffer from dementia and, of the false positives identified by the GPCOG, 38% had definite cognitive impairment but did not meet the diagnostic criteria for dementia. The GPCOG was acceptable to the general practitioners who were surveyed and was considered to be efficient in terms of time of administration. Nonetheless, the average of 6 minutes (4 minutes of direct cognitive screening and 2 minutes of informant questioning) may still be high for widespread use in general practice.

Finally, the authors of the GPCOG commend the integration of an informant component to the screening. This has the benefit of encouraging the inclusion of family members and ensuring caregiver involvement in the care planning and management of afflicted individuals. They argue that, as the general trend toward caregiver involvement increases, the opportunity to change the approach of general practitioners to the identification and management of cognitive impairment should not be lost.

Telephone cognitive screens

Telephone cognitive screens have been utilized for the identification of individuals potentially suffering from dementia. Two of the most widely used telephone screens are TICS (Telephone Interview for Cognitive Status) (Brandt et al, 1988) and TELE, a self-report interview (Gatz et al, 1995) (Tables 6.4 and 6.5). A third telephone screen was developed by Kawas et al (1995) based on the Blessed Telephone Information–Memory–Concentration Test and a fourth is known as the Minnesota Cognitive Acuity Screen (MCAS) (Knopman et al, 2000).

A study in Finland used both TELE and TICS in order to identify individuals with cognitive impairment (Jarvenpaa et al, 2002). Subjects with Alzheimer's disease were compared to healthy controls. TICS had a sensitivity of 86.7% and specificity of 88.5% while the TELE had an even higher sensitivity of 90.0% and 88.5% specificity. The ROC curves for both tests are shown in Figure 6.6. Moreover, the correlations with the

Table 6.4 Cognitive items used on the TELE (from Jarvenpaa et al, 2002, with permission from S. Karger AG).

Item	Points	Proportion of patients with correct answer (%)	Proportion of controls with correct answer (%)
Name	1	100	100
Age	1	47	100
Day and month of birth	1	90	96
Year of birth	1	83	100
Date, month, year, day of week[1], season[1]	5*	20	69
Repeating 'rose, ball, key'	1	80	96
Counting backwards from 20 by threes	3*	33	88
The current President of Finland	1	33	88
President before him	1	33	100
Recalling 'rose, ball, key'	3*	20	69
Recognition of 3 words (if miss recall)	0.5 each		
Similarities[2]: orange and banana; table and chair	2*	43	42
Total	20		

Asterisks indicate points of a completely correct answer.
[1]These questions replaced the original TELE question about address and an answer to: 'What kind of place is that?'.
[2]This question replaced the original TELE question about similarities and differences between pairs of nouns.

MMSE were high for both the TELE and TICS at 0.87 and 0.86, respectively. Jarvenpaa et al (2002) argued that telephone screens for cognitive impairment have potential use in longitudinal studies as well as for screening populations in epidemiological studies. The TELE appears to have an advantage, as it is a shorter test yet with similar psychometric properties to the longer telephone screens.

Table 6.5 Cognitive items used on the TICS (from Jarvenpaa et al, 2002, with permission from S. Karger AG).

Item	Points	Proportion of patients with correct answer (%)	Proportion of controls with correct answer (%)
Name[1]	1	100	100
Date, month, year, day of week, season	5*	20	69
The current President of Finland	1	33	88
Counting backwards from 20 to 0	2*	60	88
A 10-word list	10*	24[2]	46[2]
Counting backwards from 100 by sevens	5*	7	38
'What do people usually use to cut paper?' (1 point for 'scissors' or 'shears')			
'How many things are in a dozen?' (1 point for '12')			
'What do you call the prickly green plant that lives in the desert?' (1 point for 'cactus')	4*	43	81
'What animal does wool come from?' (1 point for 'sheep')			
'Say this: 'The pupil solved a complicated task'.			
'Say this: 'No ifs, ands or buts'.	2*	43	73
Tapping five times with finger on the part of the phone one speaks into	2*	60	92
The opposite of 'west'			
The opposite of 'generous'	2*	57	73
'Where are you right now?' (street, city, zip code, county)	4*	37	81
Total	38		

Asterisks indicate points of a completely correct answer.
Questions about house number (difficult to verify) and vice-president (does not exist in Finland) were eliminated from the original TICS protocol.
[1]This question gave 2 points (1 point for first name and 1 point for last name) on the original TICS protocol.
[2]Proportion of correct words on a 10-word list in the patient and control groups on an average.

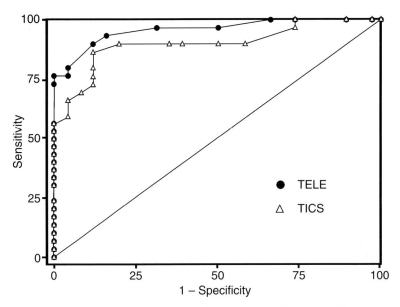

Figure 6.6 *ROC curves for telephone screens. (Reproduced from Jarvenpaa et al, 2002, with permission from S. Karger AG.)*

The most discriminating questions on the TELE and TICS telephone interviews are as follows. For TELE: orientation to time; three-word recall; and former Head of State. For TICS: serial 7's from 100; orientation to time; and current Head of State. For the MCAS the three most discriminating features were orientation; attention; and delayed word recall. Summarizing the analyses of these three telephone screens, it would appear that orientation to time, three-word recall and knowledge of the current and/or former Head of State are the most discriminating items for this type of screening.

There are limitations to telephone screening because of the significant sensory impairment, hearing and visual, in many elderly people. This method does not allow ready assessment of praxis, reading or visuospatial tasks and it cannot control for the use of aids for orientation, such as calendars and newspapers.

The MCAS (Knopman et al, 2000) used a telephone cognitive screen that consisted of nine brief tests: orientation, attention, delayed word recall, comprehension, repetition, naming, computation, judgement and verbal fluency. Experienced nurses and psychologists were able to administer this test in less than 20 minutes (*still a significant amount of time*). The optimal sensitivity and specificity was found to be 97.5% and 98.5%, respectively. However, the main limitation of this study was that it compared cognitively impaired subjects in nursing homes to healthy controls. Thus, the findings may not be generalizable to other populations.

An innovative computer-automated dementia screen uses a touch-tone telephone and an interactive voice response (IVR) system that integrates telecommunications networks with computer-automated processing (Mundt et al, 2001). The mean time to complete these calls was just over 12 minutes, significantly better than the MCAS instrument of Knopman et al (2000). Only a 10% hang-up rate was reported. The feedback from cognitively intact individuals revealed that 85% of respondents rated this system as 'easy or very easy' to use while only 7% found the system 'difficult or very difficult'. Furthermore, 76% of subjects who suffered from mild to moderate cognitive impairment reported the system as easy or very easy while only 10% indicated that it was difficult or very difficult. These are proportions not dissimilar to the intact subjects. Sensitivity and specificity in differentiating mild dementia and normals was approximately 80%.

Limitations of the IVR system include the hearing or visual impairment of subjects and the limitations posed by disabling arthritis and manipulating a telephone. The authors believe, however, that most cognitively intact senior citizens are increasingly familiar with IVR systems that are used by banks, businesses, airlines and medical clinics. They conclude that the components of a computer-automated telephone system are currently in place. This has the potential to provide dementia screening, education and referrals, as well as monitoring.

A variant of the telephone cognitive screen was used by Mintzer et al (1998) to interview caregivers. They used a caregiver telephone screen to identify care recipients who were likely to have dementia. Of the 15 subjects who ultimately agreed to a complete assessment, all were confirmed as suffering from dementia on clinical assessment. The Haycox Dementia Behaviour Scale (≥ 8) and the Blessed Dementia

Functional Sub-Scale (≥ 4) used to identify potential subjects with dementia found a very high correlation between the telephone-administered and the in-person assessments.

Conclusion

There is now a fair body of evidence to suggest that telephone cognitive screens may have a place in epidemiological studies and follow-up of longitudinal studies of cognitive impairment. Intuitively, one may feel that the telephone screen is not as valid as an in-person cognitive screen, yet the data suggest otherwise. Further testing and confirmation of these initial findings will be helpful.

References

Benton AL (1983) *Contributions to Neuropsychological Assessment*. New York: Oxford University Press.

Blessed G, Tomlinson BE, Roth M (1968) The association between qualitative measures of dementia and senile change in the cerebral grey matter of elderly subjects. *Br J Psychiatry* 114:797.

Borson S, Brush M, Gil E, Scanlan JM, Vitaliano PP et al (1999) The clock drawing test: utility for dementia detection in multi-ethnic elders. *J Gerontol Med Sci* 54A:M534–M540.

Borson S, Scanlan J, Brush M, Vitaliano P, Dokmak A (2000) The Mini-Cog: A cognitive 'vital signs' measure for dementia screening in multi-lingual elderly. *Int J Ger Psychiatry* 15:1021–1027.

Brandt J, Spenser M, Folstein M (1988) The telephone interview for cognitive status. *Neuropsychiatry Neuropsychol Behav Neurol* 45:1352–1359.

Brodaty H, Pond D, Kemp NM, Luscombe G, Harding L et al (2002) The GPCOG: A new screening test for dementia designed for general practice. *J Am Geriatr Soc* 50:530–534.

Buschke H, Kuslansky G, Katz M, Stewart WF, Sliwinski MJ et al (1999) Screening for dementia with the memory impairment screen. *Neurology* 52:231–238.

Folstein MF, Folstein SE, McHugh PR (1975) Mini-Mental State: a practical method for grading the cognitive state of patients for the clinician. *J Psychiatr Res* 12:189–198.

Froehlich TE, Robison JT, Inouye SK (1999) Screening for dementia in the out-patient setting: the time and change test. *J Am Geriatr Soc* 46:1506–1511.

Gatz M, Reynolds C, Nikolic J, Lowe B, Karel M et al (1995) An empirical test of telephone screening to identify potential dementia cases. *Int Psychogeriatr* 3:429–438.

Grober E, Buschke H, Crystal H, Bang S, Dresner R (1988) Screening for dementia by memory testing. *Neurology* **38**:900–903.

Harwood DMJ, Hope T, Jacoby R (1997) Cognitive impairment in medical inpatients. I: Screening for dementia—is history better than mental state? *Age Ageing* **26**:31–35.

Heun R, Papassotiropoulos A, Jennssen F (1998) The validity of psychometric instruments for detection of dementia in the elderly general population. *Int J Geriatr Psychiatry* **13**:368–380.

Hodkinson HM (1972) Evaluation of a mental test score for assessment of mental impairment in the elderly. *Age Ageing* **1**:233.

Inouye SK, Robison JT, Froehlich TE, Richardson ED (1998) The time and change test: A simple screening test for dementia. *J Gerontol* **53A**:M281–M286.

Isaacs B, Kennie AT (1973) The set test as an aid to the detection of dementia in old people. *Br J Psychiatry* **123**:467–470.

Jarvenpaa T, Rinne JO, Raiha I, Koskenvuo MK, Lopponen M et al (2002) Characteristics of two telephone screens for cognitive impairment. *Dement Geriatr Cogn Disord* **13**:149–155.

Jitapunkul S, Pillay I, Ebrahim S (1991) The abbreviated mental test: Its use and validity. *Age Ageing* **20**:332–336.

Jorm AF, Mackinnon AJ, Henderson AS, Scott R, Christensen H et al (1995) The Psychogeriatric Assessment Scales: A multidimensional alternative to categorical diagnoses of dementia and depression in the elderly. *Psychol Med* **25**:447–460.

Katzman R, Brown T, Fuld P, Peck A, Schechter R et al (1983) Validation of a short Orientation–Memory–Concentration Test of cognitive impairment. *Am J Psychiatry* **140**:734–739.

Kawas C, Karagiozis H, Resau L, Corrada M, Brookmeyer R (1995) Reliability of the Blessed Telephone Information–Memory–Concentration test. *J Geriatr Psychiatry Neurol* **8**:238–242.

Knopman DS, Knudson D, Yoes ME, Weiss DJ (2000) Development and standardization of a new telephone cognitive screening test: The Minnesota Cognitive Acuity Screen (MCAS). *NNBM* **13**:286–296.

Koivisto K, Helkala EL, Reinikainen KJ, Hänninen T, Mykkänen L et al (1992) Population-based dementia screening program in Kuopio: The effect of education, age, and sex on brief neuropsychological tests. *J Geriatr Psychiatry Neurol* **5**:162–171.

Kokmen E, Smith GE, Petersen RC, Tangalos E, Ivnik RC (1991) The short test of mental status. Correlations with standardised psychometric testing. *Arch Neurol* **48**:725–728.

Kuslansky G, Buschke H, Katz M, Sliwinski M, Lipton RB (2002) Screening for Alzheimer's disease: the memory impairment screen versus the conventional three-word memory test. *J Am Geriatr Soc* **50**:1086–1091.

Lawton MP, Brody EM (1969) Assessment of older people: Self-maintaining and instrumental activities of daily living. *Gerontologist* **9**:179–186.

Lorentz WJ, Scanlan JM, Borson S (2002) Brief screening tests for dementia. *Can J Psychiatry* **47(8)**:723–733.

Mintzer J, Nietert P, Costa K, Rust P, Hoerning K (1998) Identifying persons with dementia by use of a caregiver telephone interview. *Am J Geriatr Psychiatry* **6**:176–179.

Monsch AU, Siefritz E, Taylor KI, Ermini-Funfschilling D, Stahelin HB et al (1997) Category fluency is also predominantly affected in Swiss Alzheimer's disease patients. *Acta Neurol Scand* **95**:81–84.

Morris JC, Heyman A, Mohs RC, Hughes JP, van Belle G et al (1989) The consortium to establish a registry for Alzheimer's disease (CERAD). Part I. Clinical and neuropsychological assessment of Alzheimer's disease. *Neurology* **39**:1159–1165.

Mundt JC, Ferber KL, Rizzo M, Greist JH (2001) Computer-automated dementia screening using a touch-tone telephone. *Arch Intern Med* **161**:2481–2487.

Oswald WD, Roth E (1978) *Der Zahlen-Verbindungs-Test (ZVT)*. Hogrefe, Göttingen: Verlag für Psychologie, 1–58.

Reitan R (1958) Validity of the trail making test as an indicator of organic brain damage. *Percept Motor Skills* **8**:271–276.

Roth M, Tym E, Mountjoy CQ, Huppert FA, Hendrie H et al (1986) CAMDEX: A standardised instrument for the diagnosis of mental disorder in the elderly with special reference to the early detection of dementia. *Br J Psychiatry* **149**: 698–709.

Royall DR (2000) Executive cognitive impairment: A novel perspective on dementia. *Neuroepidemiology* **19**:293–299.

Scanlan J, Borson S (2001) The Mini-Cog: Receiver operating characteristics with expert and naïve raters. *Int J Geriatr Psychiatry* **16**:216–222.

Shulman KI (2000) Clock-drawing: Is it the ideal cognitive screening test? *Int J Geriatr Psychiatry* **15**:548–561.

Solomon PR, Hirschoff A, Kelly B, Relin M, Brush M et al (1998) A 7 minute neurocognitive screening battery highly sensitive to Alzheimer's disease. *Arch Neurol* **55**:349–355.

Teng EL, Hasegawa K, Homma A, Imai Y, Larson E et al (1994) The Cognitive Abilities Screening Instrument (CASI): a practical test for cross-cultural epidemiological studies of dementia. *Int Psychogeriatr* **6**:45–58.

Appendix 6.1

Mental Test Score (reproduced from Hodkinson, 1972, with permission from Oxford University Press).

	Score
Name	0/1
Age	0/1
Time (to nearest hour)	0/1
Time of day	0/1
Name and address for five-minute recall; this should be repeated by the patient to ensure that it has been heard correctly.	
Mr. John Brown	0/1/2
42 West Street	0/1/2
Gateshead	0/1
Day of week	0/1
Date (correct day of month)	0/1

Month	0/1
Year	0/1
Place: type of place (i.e. hospital)	0/1
Name of hospital	0/1
Name of ward	0/1
Name of town	0/1
Recognition of two persons (doctor, nurse, etc.)	0/1/2
Date of birth (day and month sufficient)	0/1
Place of birth (town)	0/1
School attended	0/1
Former occupation	0/1
Name of wife, sib or next of kin	0/1
Date of First World War (year sufficient)	0/1
Date of Second World War (date sufficient)	0/1
Name of present Monarch	0/1
Name of present Prime Minister	0/1
Months of year backwards	0/1/2
Count 1–20	0/1/2
Count 20–1	0/1/2
Total	(34)

Appendix 6.2

Abbreviated Mental Test Score. Each question scores one point (reproduced from Hodkinson, 1972, with permission from Oxford University Press).

1. Age
2. Time (to nearest hour)
3. Address for recall at end of test – this should be repeated by the patient to ensure that it has been heard correctly:
    42 West Street
4. Year
5. Name of hospital
6. Recognition of two persons (doctor, nurse, etc.)
7. Date of birth
8. Year of First World War
9. Name of present Monarch
10. Count backwards 20–1

Appendix 6.3

GPCOG Patient Examination. Unless specified, each question should be asked only once (reproduced from Brodaty et al, 2002, with permission from Blackwell Science).

Name and address for subsequent recall test

1. 'I am going to give you a name and address. After I have said it, I want you to repeat it. Remember this name and address because I am going to ask you to tell me again in a few minutes: John Brown, 42 West Street, Kensington.' (Allow a maximum of four attempts but do not score yet)

	Correct	Incorrect
Time orientation		
2. What is the date? (exact only)	☐	☐
Clock drawing (visuospatial functioning) – use page with printed circle		
3. Please mark in all the numbers to indicate the hours of a clock (correct spacing required)	☐	☐
4. Please mark in hands to show 10 minutes past eleven o'clock (11:10)	☐	☐
5. Can you tell me something that happened in the news recently? (recently = in the past week)	☐	☐
Recall		
6. What was the name and address I asked you to remember?		
John	☐	☐
Brown	☐	☐
42	☐	☐
West (St)	☐	☐
Kensington	☐	☐

Scoring guidelines

Clock drawing: For a correct response to question 3, the numbers 12, 3, 6 and 9 should be in the correct quadrants of the circle and the other numbers should be approximately correctly placed. For a correct response to question 4, the hands should be pointing to the 11 and the 2, but the respondent should not be penalized for failure to distinguish the long and short hands.

Information: Respondents are not required to provide extensive details, as long as they demonstrate awareness of a recent news story. If a general answer is given, such as 'war', 'a lot of rain', ask for details – if unable to give details, the answer should be scored as incorrect.

GPCOG Informant Interview
Ask the informant: 'Compared to a few years ago,

		Yes	No	Don't know	N/A
I.	Does the patient have more trouble remembering things that have happened recently?	☐	☐	☐	☐
II.	Does he or she have more trouble recalling conversations a few days later?	☐	☐	☐	☐
III.	When speaking, does the patient have more difficulty in finding the right word or tend to use the wrong words more often?	☐	☐	☐	☐
IV.	Is the patient less able to manage money and financial affairs (e.g. paying bills, budgeting)?	☐	☐	☐	☐
V.	Is the patient less able to manage his or her medication independently?	☐	☐	☐	☐
VI.	Does the patient need more assistance with transport (either private or public)?	☐	☐	☐	☐

chapter 7

Informant questionnaires

Because of the nature of dementias and neuropsychiatric disorders, it is highly desirable (if not essential) to have the perspective of a reliable informant in assessing cognition. Moreover, dementia involves a deterioration or decline in cognitive ability from a premorbid level (Jorm and Jacomb, 1989). Because there is a risk of both false-positive and false-negative assessments based on premorbid IQ and education, it is necessary to have an estimate of the premorbid level of cognitive ability. Individuals who have always been limited in intellectual ability may be falsely diagnosed as demented while highly intelligent and educated individuals could be misclassified as intact despite the fact that they have sustained a substantial cognitive decline (Jorm and Jacomb, 1989). Cognitive decline was estimated by using informants who had knowledge of the subject's premorbid level of functioning and behavior. Informant reports were postulated to have greater validity, because their observations were based on the performance on independent activities of daily living rather than investigator-initiated cognitive tests.

IQCODE

The original test developed by Jorm and Jacomb (1989) is known as the IQCODE (the Informant Questionnaire on Cognitive Decline in the Elderly). This is a 26-item questionnaire in which informants are asked to rate the degree of change over a 10-year period related to various aspects of an elderly person's memory and intelligence (Jorm and Korten, 1988). The informants are asked to rate the subject's performance on a scale ranging from 'much better' to 'much worse'. The psychometric properties of this instrument indicated that the IQCODE measured a broad general factor of cognitive decline. Moreover, it had high internal consistency (Jorm and Jacomb, 1989) as well as high test–retest reliability that included retesting within a few days ($r = 0.96$) as well as retesting over a period of a year ($r = 0.75$) (Jorm and Jacomb, 1989; Jorm et al, 1991). As a measure of its independence from premorbid intelligence and ability, the IQCODE showed virtually no correlation with the subject's education or occupational status. Similarly, the IQCODE has also been found to have a poor correlation with the performance on the National Adult Reading Test (NART), a measure of premorbid intelligence (Jorm et al, 1991).

The validity of the IQCODE has been measured with a variety of standards including correlation with the Mini Mental State Examination (MMSE) (Bowers et al, 1990). The predictive validity of the IQCODE was substantiated in part on the assumption that a severe dementia would increase the probability of institutionalization. Indeed, dementing subjects who eventually were moved into residential care were found to have worse scores than dementing subjects who remained in the community (Jorm and Jacomb, 1989).

In a subsequent analysis, Jorm (1994) determined that a shorter 16-item form of the IQCODE performed as well as the original 26-item questionnaire (Table 7.1). Data from four studies were used to assess the psychometric properties of the original 26 IQCODE items. Individual items were assessed in terms of item–total correlations, test–retest reliabilities, correlations with indicators of current cognitive functioning and correlations with indicators of premorbid cognitive functioning. Similar to the original IQCODE, items on the shorter version were relatively uninfluenced by education. Moreover, the item selection process used by Jorm selected out items that were sensitive to cognitive changes at the milder end of the cognitive spectrum. Therefore, the short-form items were more likely to detect early decline rather than discriminating

Table 7.1 The Informant Questionnaire on Cognitive Decline in the Elderly (IQCODE) (reproduced from Jorm, 1994, with permission from Cambridge University Press).

Now we want you to remember what your friend or relative was like 10 years ago and to compare it with what he/she is like now. 10 years ago was in 19___ Below are situations where this person has to use his/her memory or intelligence and we want you to indicate whether this has improved, stayed the same, or got worse in that situation over the past 10 years. Note the importance of comparing his/her present performance *with 10 years ago*. So if 10 years ago this person always forgot where he/she had left things, and he/she still does, then this would be considered 'Hasn't changed much'. Please indicate the changes you have observed by *circling the appropriate answer.*

Compared with 10 years ago how is this person at:

	1	2	3	4	5
1. Recognizing the faces of family and friends	Much improved	A bit improved	Not much change	A bit worse	Much worse
2. Remembering the names of family and friends	Much improved	A bit improved	Not much change	A bit worse	Much worse
3. *Remembering things about family and friends, e.g. occupations, birthdays, addresses	Much improved	A bit improved	Not much change	A bit worse	Much worse
4. *Remembering things that have happened recently	Much improved	A bit improved	Not much change	A bit worse	Much worse
5. *Recalling conversations a few days later	Much improved	A bit improved	Not much change	A bit worse	Much worse
6. Forgetting what s/he wanted to say in the conversation	Much improved	A bit improved	Not much change	A bit worse	Much worse

Table 7.1 Continued

	1	2	3	4	5
7. *Remembering her/his address and telephone number	Much improved	A bit improved	Not much change	A bit worse	Much worse
8. *Remembering what day and month it is	Much improved	A bit improved	Not much change	A bit worse	Much worse
9. *Remembering where things are usually kept	Much improved	A bit improved	Not much change	A bit worse	Much worse
10. * Remembering where to find things which have been put in a different place from usual	Much improved	A bit improved	Not much change	A bit worse	Much worse
11. Adjusting to any change in her/his day-to-day routine	Much improved	A bit improved	Not much change	A bit worse	Much worse
12. *Knowing how to work familiar machines around the house	Much improved	A bit improved	Not much change	A bit worse	Much worse
13. *Learning to use a new gadget or machine around the house	Much improved	A bit improved	Not much change	A bit worse	Much worse
14. *Learning new things in general	Much improved	A bit improved	Not much change	A bit worse	Much worse
15. Remembering things that happened to her/him when s/he was young	Much improved	A bit improved	Not much change	A bit worse	Much worse
16. Remembering things s/he learned when s/he was young	Much improved	A bit improved	Not much change	A bit worse	Much worse

Table 7.1 Continued

	1	2	3	4	5
17. Understanding the meaning of unusual words	Much improved	A bit improved	Not much change	A bit worse	Much worse
18. Understanding magazine or newspaper articles	Much improved	A bit improved	Not much change	A bit worse	Much worse
19. *Following a story in a book or on TV	Much improved	A bit improved	Not much change	A bit worse	Much worse
20. Composing a letter to friends or for business purposes	Much improved	A bit improved	Not much change	A bit worse	Much worse
21. Knowing about important historical events of the past	Much improved	A bit improved	Not much change	A bit worse	Much worse
22. *Making decisions on everyday matters	Much improved	A bit improved	Not much change	A bit worse	Much worse
23. *Handling money for shopping	Much improved	A bit improved	Not much change	A bit worse	Much worse
24. *Handling financial matters, e.g. the pension, dealing with the bank	Much improved	A bit improved	Not much change	A bit worse	Much worse
25. *Handling other everyday arithmetic problems e.g. knowing how much food to buy, knowing how long between visits from family or friends	Much improved	A bit improved	Not much change	A bit worse	Much worse

Table 7.1 Continued

	1	2	3	4	5
26. *Using his/her intelligence to understand what's going on and to reason things through	Much improved	A bit improved	Not much change	A bit worse	Much worse

* Items used in the short form.

Note: As administered in the studies reported here, the IQCODE was preceded by questions on sociodemographic characteristics and other aspects of the subject's health. The rating scale above has been modified to use the word 'improved' in place of 'better' in order to avoid misinterpretation.

among more severely demented individuals. However, this is precisely the use for which this test was designed. The fact that the IQCODE is likely to be used in conjunction with other questionnaires and tests (see below), makes the short version highly desirable.

In a direct comparison, the MMSE and the IQCODE were found to be equally efficient screening measures for dementia (Mulligan et al, 1996) (Figure 7.1). The MMSE was found once again to be significantly affected by low educational attainment, but the IQCODE was not affected in the same way. This study reinforced the comparability of cognitive testing and informant reports as a way of screening for dementia in clinical settings.

Jorm (1997) performed a meta-analysis on ten studies that compared an informant questionnaire with a brief cognitive test as a screen for dementia. Of the ten studies, seven used the IQCODE as the informant questionnaire in a direct comparison to the MMSE. The weighted mean effectiveness for the informant questionnaire was 1.74 (1.39–2.09) compared to the brief cognitive test, which had a weighted mean effective

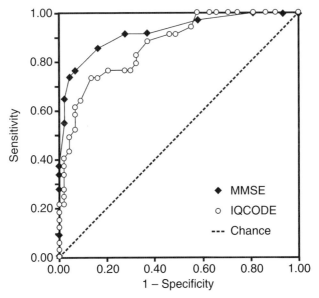

Figure 7.1 *ROC curves for dementia screening with the MMSE and IQCODE. (Reproduced from Mulligan et al, 1996, with permission from the American Medical Association.)*

ness of 1.48 (1.23–1.73). Sensitivity and specificity were 0.86 and 0.80 for the informant questionnaire and 0.79 and 0.80 for the brief cognitive test.

In short, the most commonly used informant questionnaire, the IQCODE, performed as well as the most commonly used cognitive screening test, the MMSE.

DECO (Détérioration Cognitive Observée)

Ritchie and Fuhrer (1996) validated an informant screening test using a randomly selected sample from community dwelling elderly in Bordeaux, France. The expectation was that the nature of the sample would yield a more heterogeneous range of cognitive abilities and thereby provide a higher standard for screening test validation. Thus, adjustments in cut-off points according to the predictive prevalence rate in a specific population are necessary to maintain comparable positive and negative predictive values.

The DECO is a 19-item Likert scale which covers changes in behavior including activity level, semantic and visual memory, memory for places, events and procedures, visuospatial performance and new skill learning. The informant is defined as a person who has had at least monthly contact with an elderly person for a minimum of 3 years. Each item on the scale is rated from 0 to 2. A maximum score of 38 indicates no change in behavior over the past year whereas a score of zero implies a dramatic change on all items. The optimum cut-off point was determined at 30/29, yielding 90% specificity and 89% sensitivity. The main limitation of this, instrument, like the IQCODE, is the disadvantage of any informant questionnaire – that it is applicable only to conditions that show deterioration. However, as a clinical screening instrument, this is not a restrictive condition (Appendix 7.1).

Law and Wolfson (1995) provide a lucid discussion of the advantages and limitations of informant questionnaires. This approach relies on an informant's perception of the day-to-day activities of the subject which appears to provide a more thorough and overall assessment than specific screening tests such as the MMSE. Unlike the MMSE, the IQCODE is not vulnerable to making false-positive predictions in subjects with low education. In the French version of the IQCODE, there was also no correlation between level of education and the informant scores. Therefore, the IQCODE may be useful in epidemiological studies in socially and educationally underprivileged communities.

It has been suggested that, in dementia, the impairment of 'active and effortful information processing' precedes that of 'automatic information processing'. Hence, the IQCODE's emphasis on the assessment of active information processing allows this scale to discriminate between mild dementia and normal aging in a way that is different from some screening tests. The items in the IQCODE are specifically geared in this direction, for example in the assessment of ability to learn new things, the recall of recent events and making decisions regarding money.

The IQCODE is effective and relatively inexpensive to administer. It is a self-administered questionnaire and can be done while the informant is waiting for their relative to be assessed or examined. It also highlights the importance of the informant not only in the diagnostic process but also in the entire management of dementia. The fact that Law and Wolfson (1995) confirmed the validity of the French version in Quebec suggests that it may be universally valid. This line of research is highlighted by the IQCODE, the DECO and the family interview component of the Cambridge Examination for Mental Disorders in the Elderly (CAMDEX) (O'Connor, 1990).

Combining cognitive testing and informant reports

Mackinnon and Mulligan (1998) demonstrated that the combination of cognitive screening using the MMSE and the short form of the IQCODE resulted in more accurate predictions of caseness than either test alone. They demonstrated that the informant report could be readily incorporated into the assessment for dementia and thus increase the accuracy of detection of cases and non-cases.

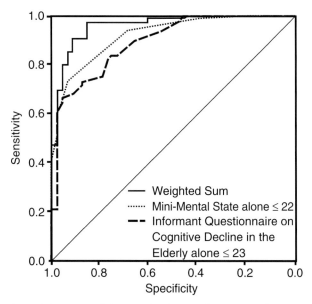

Figure 7.2 *ROC curves of the weighted sum of scores on the IQCODE and MMSE. (Reproduced from MacKinnon and Mulligan, 1998, with permission from the American Psychiatric Association. http://AJP.psychiatryonline.org)*

A combination approach is based on the assumption that informant reports and cognitive tests do not measure the same attributes. Because cognitive testing is influenced by education and premorbid intelligence while informant questionnaires are not, they make for a natural comple-ment to a screening battery. Moreover, scores on the informant ques-tionnaires can be influenced by the affective state of the informant and the nature of the relationship between the patient and informant. Therefore, the combination approach does seem to have face validity. The receiver operating characteristic (ROC) curves for this study are shown in Figure 7.2 and the psychometric properties in Table 7.2. The area under the curve of 0.96 (0.92–0.99) for the combined IQCODE and MMSE was significantly greater than the area under the curve of either test alone.

This 'combination' study was carried out in a clinical population whose psychometric performance (including sensitivity and specificity) is significantly influenced by the nature of the population being

Table 7.2 Performance of Mini Mental State Examination, Informant Questionnaire on Cognitive Decline in the Elderly and test combinations as screens for dementia in 106 elderly patients (reproduced from Mackinnon and Mulligan, 1998, with permission from The American Psychiatric Association. http://AJP.psychiatryonline.org).

Test and Score for Diagnosis of Dementia	Sensitivity		Specificity		Positive predictive value		Negative predictive value	
	Index	95% Confidence Interval	Index	95% Confidence Interval	Index	95% Confidence Interval	Index	95% Confidence Interval
Individual tests								
Mini Mental State score ≤ 23	0.76	0.63–0.86	0.90	0.77–0.97	0.90	0.78–0.97	0.75	0.62–0.86
Mini Mental State score ≤ 26	0.95	0.86–0.99	0.60	0.45–0.74	0.74	0.63–0.84	0.91	0.75–0.98
Informant report score ≥ 3.6	0.90	0.79–0.96	0.65	0.49–0.78	0.75	0.64–0.85	0.84	0.68–0.94
'Or' rule — Mini Mental State score ≤ 23 or informant report score > 4.00	0.93	0.83–0.98	0.81	0.67–0.91	0.86	0.75–0.93	0.91	0.78–0.97
'And' rule — Mini Mental State score ≤ 25 and informant report score ≥ 3.62	0.86	0.75–0.94	0.85	0.72–0.94	0.88	0.76–0.95	0.84	0.70–0.93
Weighted sum for various probabilities of caseness[a]								
Pr (case) ≥ 0.40 (−0.40)	0.97	0.88–1.00	0.85	0.72–0.94	0.89	0.78–0.95	0.95	0.84–0.99
Pr (case) ≥ 0.50 (0.00)	0.93	0.83–0.98	0.85	0.72–0.94	0.89	0.78–0.95	0.91	0.79–0.98
Pr (case) ≥ 0.60 (0.39)	0.90	0.79–0.96	0.92	0.80–0.98	0.93	0.83–0.98	0.88–	0.76–0.95

[a] See text for calculation of Pr (case).

sampled. Therefore, it will be important to confirm that the combination approach is also superior in general population samples. From a practical perspective, adding an informant report adds little to the burden of clinicians and clinical services. It is self-administered and can be completed by mail or while the informant is waiting for the subject to be examined.

Lorentz et al (2002) concluded that informant-based tools could be as effective as cognitive instruments for dementia screening and had advantages that include longitudinal change, the focus on everyday cognitive abilities and their cross-cultural capacity. They noted that the short IQCODE took an average of 10–12 minutes (range 8–15) to administer.

In a study of Thai elderly (Senanarong et al, 2001), three questions on the IQCODE were found to carry the greatest power in classifying cognitive status. They were: (1) learning to use new gadgets; (2) knowing the day and month; and (3) handling everyday arithmetic problems. This highlights the focus of the informant questionnaires on active new learning and instrumental activities of daily living. Cross-cultural validity is highlighted by the IQCODE results in Chinese (Fuh et al, 1995); Japanese (White et al, 1994); and Spanish (Morales et al, 1995) versions in addition to the French (France) version described above (Ritchie and Fuhrer, 1996).

Lorentz et al (2002) suggested that a promising line of investigation was the further reduction of items in the informant questionnaires to create an 'ultra short IQCODE' that would contain only the essential items necessary for the detection of dementia. The work with the Thai elderly suggests that as few as three items may be sufficient, but this needs to be replicated.

References

Bowers J, Jorm AF, Henderson S, Harris P (1990) General practitioners' detection of depression and dementia in elderly patients. *Med J Aust* **153**:192–196.
Fuh JL, Teng EL, Lin KN, Larson EB, Wang SJ et al (1995) The Informant Questionnaire on Cognitive Decline in the Elderly (IQCODE) as a screening

tool for dementia for a predominant illiterate Chinese population. *Neurology* **45**:92–96.

Jorm AF (1994) A short form of the Informant Questionnaire on Cognitive Decline in the Elderly (IQCODE): development and cross-validation. *Psychol Med* **24**:145–153.

Jorm AF (1997) Methods of screening for dementia: A meta-analysis of studies comparing an informant questionnaire with a brief cognitive test. *Alzheimer Dis Assoc Disord* **11(3)**:158–162.

Jorm AF, Jacomb PA (1989) The Informant Questionnaire on Cognitive Decline in the Elderly (IQCODE): socio-demographic correlates, reliability, validity and some norms. *Psychol Med* **19**:1015–1022.

Jorm AF, Korten AE (1988) Assessment of cognitive decline in the elderly by informant interview. *Br J Psychiatry* **152**:209–213.

Jorm AF, Scott R, Cullen JS, Mackinnon AJ (1991) Performance of the Informant Questionnaire on Cognitive Decline in the Elderly (IQCODE) as a screening test for dementia. *Psychol Med* **21**:785–790.

Law S, Wolfson C (1995) Validation of a French version of an informant-based questionnaire as a screening test for Alzheimer's Disease. *Br J Psychiatry* **167**:541–544.

Lorentz WJ, Scanlan JM, Borson S (2002) Brief screening tests for dementia. *Can J Psychiatry* **47(8)**:723–733.

Mackinnon A, Mulligan R (1998) Combining cognitive testing and informant report to increase accuracy in screening for dementia. *Am J Psychiatry* **155**:1529–1535.

Morales J-M, Gonzalez-Montalvo J-I, Bermejo F, Del-Ser T (1995) The screening of mild dementia with a shortened Spanish version of the 'Informant Questionnaire on Cognitive Decline in the Elderly'. *Alzheimer Dis Assoc Disord* **9**:105–111.

Mulligan R, Mackinnon A, Jorm AF, Giannakopulos P, Michel J-P (1996) A comparison of alternative methods of screening for dementia in clinical settings. *Arch Neurol* **53**:532–536.

O'Connor DW (1990) The contribution of CAMDEX to the diagnosis of mild dementia in community surveys. *Psychiatr J Univ Ottawa* **15**:216–220.

Ritchie K, Fuhrer R (1996) The validation of an informant screening test for irreversible cognitive decline in the elderly: performance characteristics within a general population sample. *Int J Geriatr Psychiatry* **11**:149–156.

Senanarong V, Assavisaraporn S, Sivasiriyanonds N, Printarakul T, Jamjumrus P et al (2001) The IQCODE: an alternative screening test for dementia for low educated Thai elderly. *J Med Assoc Thai* **84**:648–655.

White LR, Ross GW, Petrovitch H, Masaki KH, Chiu D et al (1994) Estimation of the sensitivity and specificity of a dementia screening test in a population-based survey. *Neurobiol Aging* **15**:S42.

Appendix 7.1

(Questionnaire reproduced with permission from Ritchie and Fuhrer, 1996, with permission from John Wiley & Sons Ltd.

We would like you to tell us how your relative was a year ago. The following questions ask about a number of everyday situations. We would like you to tell us whether in these situations he/she is doing about the same, not as well or much worse, than a year ago. Put a cross in the square to show your reply.

	Better or about the same	Not as well	Much worse
Does he/she remember as well as before which day of the week and which month it is?	☐	☐	☐
When he/she goes out of the house, does he/she know the way as well as before?	☐	☐	☐
Have there been changes in his/her ability to remember his/her own address or telephone number?	☐	☐	☐
In the house, does he/she remember as well as before where things are usually kept?	☐	☐	☐
And when an object isn't in its usual place, is he/she capable of finding it again?	☐	☐	☐
In comparison with a year ago, how well is he/she able to use household appliances (washing maching, etc.....)?	☐	☐	☐
Has his/her ability to dress or undress changed at all?	☐	☐	☐
How well does he/she manage his/her money, for example doing the shopping?	☐	☐	☐
Apart from difficulties due to physical problems, has there been a reduction in his/her activity level?	☐	☐	☐

	Better or about the same	Not as well	Much worse
How well can he/she follow a story on television, in a book or told by someone?	☐	☐	☐
And writing letters for business or to friends, does he/she do this as well as a year ago?	☐	☐	☐
How well does he/she recall a conversation you have had with him/her a few days ago? Has this changed over the past year?	☐	☐	☐
And if you remind him/her of this conversation, does he/she still have difficulty remembering it in comparison with a year ago?	☐	☐	☐
Does he/she forget what he/she wanted to say in the middle of a conversation? Has this changed over the past year?	☐	☐	☐
In a conversation, does he/she sometimes have difficulty finding the right word?	☐	☐	☐
In comparison with a year ago, how well does he/she recognize the faces of people he/she knows well?	☐	☐	☐
And how well does he/she remember the names of these people?	☐	☐	☐
In comparison with a year ago, how well does he/she remember other details concerning people he/she knows well: where they live, what they do?	☐	☐	☐
Over the past year, have there been changes in his/her ability to remember what has happened recently?	☐	☐	☐

chapter 8

Neuroimaging correlates of cognitive dysfunction

It is a common misconception that neuropsychological testing alone will furnish a diagnosis. Rather, it is one part of a patient's work-up that begins with a history, physical examination including neurological assessment and mental state assessment. Only once these have been completed, and depending on the findings, should a patient be sent for investigation. It is here that the results of a neuropsychological evaluation may be enhanced by neuroimaging.

For the purposes of this chapter, neuroimaging will be broadly divided into structural and functional. The former encompasses computerized axial tomography (CT) scanning and magnetic resonance imaging (MRI), while the latter will focus on single photon emission computerized tomography (SPECT). Our decision in choosing these three imaging modalities is based on a recognition that clinicians generally have ready access to them, waiting lists aside. Other useful imaging techniques, such as functional MRI (fMRI) and positron emission tomography (PET) are largely research-based and, while their clinical utility is likely to be considerable, routine patient use is not yet established.

As a way of demonstrating the utility of neuroimaging as a clinical adjunct, a series of case reports is presented, each highlighting a particular aspect of the imaging spectrum.

Case report 1

A 44-year-old married man, riding his motorbike, was struck by a car. He lost consciousness for approximately 10 minutes. On arrival at the hospital emergency room, his Glasgow Coma Scale (GCS) score was noted as 13. There were no other injuries other than his closed head injury and he was admitted to a trauma ward. His post-traumatic amnesia lasted between 36 and 48 hours. A brain CT scan was normal (Figure 8.1).

Background information revealed that he owned a picture-framing business together with a partner. His first marriage had ended in divorce while he was in his early twenties. He had remarried 10 years back and had a 7-year-old son. He had a number of close friends and an active, happy social life.

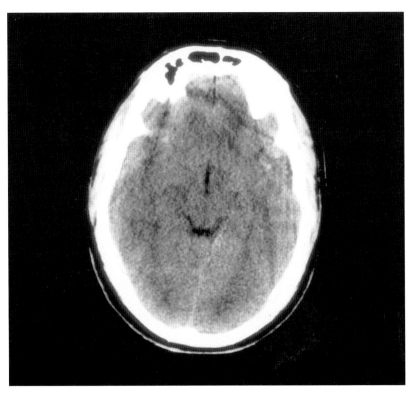

Figure 8.1 *Normal CT brain scan in a 44-year-old man with behavioral changes following traumatic brain injury.*

After a 3-day hospital admission, he was discharged home and advised to rest for a week before returning for a follow-up appointment with the hospital's traumatic brain injury clinic. He kept his appointment, accompanied by his wife, who appeared agitated and asked to speak with the doctor alone. The patient agreed to this, although he expressed surprise at the need for secrecy.

Once alone with the clinic's staff, his wife recounted a tale of mayhem at home. Her husband was unrecognizable from the man she married. The biggest problem was his unprovoked, explosive outbursts of rage. These occurred a couple of times each day, were impossible to predict and frightening to witness. Although he had not resorted to physical violence, his shouting and verbally threatening behavior had frightened both her and their son. The boy had taken to avoiding his father and would cower in his presence. Furthermore, she had become aware of a new-found impulsivity in her husband's behavior, this impetuosity frequently associated with poor judgement and bellicosity. Thus, despite a recommendation from the hospital staff that he take time off work to recuperate, he had returned to his framing shop the day after discharge. His behavior towards customers was impatient and rudely provocative, and more than one disgruntled customer had fled the store promising never to return. This in turn had led to arguments between her husband and his business partner, who had also taken exception to the unnecessarily rude behavior. As with the temper outbursts, the patient expressed amazement at the depth of feeling and distress his behavior had engendered in others, although he did acknowledge he was not his 'usual self'. He described his mood as 'up and down'.

The patient was once again advised to take time off work. He was started on carbamazepine for his aggression and a series of investigations, including brain MRI with gradient echo sequences and brain SPECT, were booked. However, within days his wife phoned the clinic complaining that the situation at home was untenable. The precipitant for her distressed call was an incident at their son's weekly soccer game, where her husband had become irate and provoked an altercation with the referee. Other parents had come to the defence of the official and her husband had been assaulted by another parent. The children had found the episode upsetting and the game had to be abandoned. The patient's son was now refusing to return and play for his team, an activity that had always been one of his favorite sports.

The patient's wife, and another family member who had also phoned in to express concern, were both adamant that the aggressive behavior represented a dramatic departure from his premorbid personality characteristics. Prior to his accident, the patient was described as hard-working and diligent while attentive and caring as a father. His wife readily admitted he had been somewhat dependent on her, both emotionally and with respect to running the household, but he had never been violent and had never raised his voice to their son. The paroxysms of rage were unlike anything she had experienced during their 10 years together.

As for the patient, the episode at the soccer match had been upsetting and convinced him that something was wrong with his behavior. He was able to detect the fear his presence engendered in his son and that left him feeling guilty and remorseful. Despite this new level of insight, he professed an inability to control his outbursts of rage. Throughout the verbal conflagrations, he was aware of what was going on and realized that some of his remarks were inappropriate. He, too, was beginning to find his lack of control frightening. In order to defuse the atmosphere of crisis that had developed at home, the patient was admitted to a neuropsychiatry inpatient service.

Apart from intermittent agitation, his mental state was unremarkable. At times he would appear tetchy with the nursing staff, but the explosions of rage were not witnessed. Mood was described as a little low, but seemed appropriate to his current difficult social situation. Classic depressive cognitive distortions were not present. A Mini Mental State Examination (MMSE) (Folstein et al, 1975) gave a score of 29/30. Neuropsychological testing was booked for 3 months post-injury. Neuroimaging was, however, undertaken while he was an inpatient and was grossly abnormal. A standard spin echo MRI scan was normal, but on the gradient echo sequence, multiple hemosiderin deposits, indicative of axonal shearing and microhemorrhages, were discernible, particularly in orbitofrontal and anterior temporal regions (Figure 8.2). These findings of structural brain abnormalities were in turn confluent with the SPECT data, for the functional brain imaging revealed hypoperfusion in the vicinity of the hemosiderin deposits (Figure 8.3).

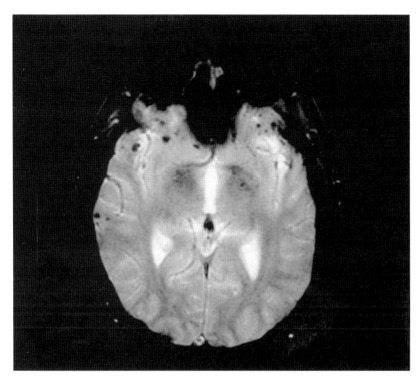

Figure 8.2 *Abnormal gradient echo MRI scan showing scattered hemosiderin deposits in anterior temporal and inferior frontal regions. The patient's CT scan (Figure 8.1) was normal.*

Over the course of the next few months, various combinations of psychotropic medications were tried to reduce his aggression. Results were only partially successful, with the most beneficial regime proving to be olanzapine 2.5 mg per day, fluoxetine 10 mg per day and carbamazepine 400 mg twice daily. Neuropsychological testing revealed mild deficits on tests of attention and short-term memory, with scores still falling in the normal range. While these represented a decline in performance relative to premorbid intellectual levels, there remained a dramatic discrepancy between his relatively intact neuropsychological profile and his marked behavioral disturbance. This was explained by his cerebral pathology impacting largely on the orbitofrontal cortex, where deficits on standard neuropsychological paradigms are often not discernible. The patient was therefore tested in our research laboratory, where the 'Gambling' task

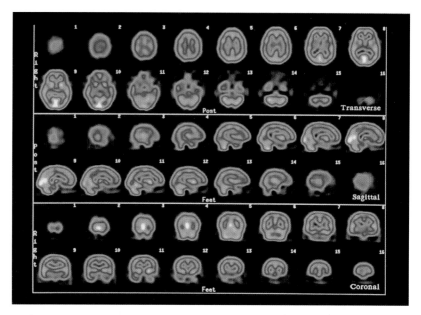

Figure 8.3 *Abnormal brain SPECT scan showing areas of hypoperfusion in medial orbitofrontal areas compatible with hemosiderin deposits seen on gradient echo MRI.*

(Bechara et al, 1994) was administered. His performance here was grossly impaired, displaying a marked impulsivity and an inability to monitor and check responses that were clearly disadvantageous. Finally, subtle olfactory deficits were noted on the 40-item University of Pennsylvania Smell Identification Test (Doty, 1983). Bringing all the clinical, neuropsychological and neuroimaging data together, a DSM-IV diagnosis of personality change due to a general medical condition, i.e. a traumatic brain injury, was made. In the months that ensued, the man's picture-framing business went into liquidation and his friendship with his business partner ended, the latter bitterly blaming our patient's erratic and extreme behavior for their loss of clientele. Our patient's marriage endured but only with extensive supportive therapy for his spouse, while his son, too, needed counseling.

This case contains a number of points of singular interest. First, from a clinical perspective is the relative insensitivity of the GCS in predicting behavioral outcome. A GCS score of 13 places the injury in the mild category, which by definition is limited to GCS scores from 13 to 15. A suggestion that the injury may have been more severe comes from his post-traumatic amnesia that exceeded 24 hours. However, there was little from these two indices that pointed towards such a poor outcome.

The second point of interest was the absence of cerebral pathology on brain CT. Only once the brain MRI scan was done, did the hemosiderin deposits show up on the gradient echo sequence. While CT of the brain is useful in traumatic brain injury, revealing an array of pathology from skull fracture to subdural, extradural and intracerebral hemorrhages, it lacks sensitivity in revealing the signs of diffuse axonal injury.

The third notable feature was the paucity of gross deficits on conventional neuropsychiatric testing that included such staples as the Wechsler Intelligence Scales (Wechsler, 1981), California Verbal Learning Test (Delis et al, 1987), Wisconsin Card Sort Test (Heaton, 1981) and the Paced Auditory Serial Addition Task (Gronwall, 1977). The ability of patients with primarily orbitofrontal deficits to perform within normal parameters on these tests has been described (Damasio, 1994) and may give the misleading impression that all is well, cognitively. Only when the functional integrity of this region is probed with more experimental paradigms do deficits emerge.

One practical consideration of these three points is that the mild GCS score, normal brain CT and few 'conventional' neuropsychological deficits led many of the patient's health-care providers and the insurance industry to deem his injury inconsequential and his aggressive outbursts the product of 'acting out' behavior allied to long-standing characterological issues. Not only was this assessment incorrect, for there was little on history to suggest this man had an abnormal premorbid personality, but mis-attributing the behavior in such a pejorative fashion added to the patient's (and family's) burden by heightening their sense of frustration in coming to terms with his significant neuropsychiatric morbidity. Only once the results of the MRI, SPECT, UPSIT and 'Gambling' Test were explained to the family and caregivers did this situation improve. His insurance company, however, remained harder to convince, in part because of the industry's universal fixation with the

GCS as the single arbiter of injury severity. This inability to look beyond this oversimplification ensured an on-going dispute between the patient and his main source of income after the accident, namely his disability settlement. This adversarial relationship was a perpetual source of annoyance to a man whose personality change left him poorly equipped to deal with stressors of this nature.

From a neuropsychiatric perspective, the case is a good illustration that confluence of findings; clinical, radiological and neuropsychological, can help explain such profound disability. Our patient did not have an iron bar driven through his skull as happened to the unfortunate Mr Phineas Gage (Appendix 8.1), but his brain damage was confined to similar anatomical areas and his clinical presentation characterized by impulsivity and poor social judgement overlapped with his medically famous predecessor.

Case report 2

A 50-year-old man was brought by the police to the Emergency Room. The police had initially arrested him on High Street where his unsteady gait had resembled that of a drunk. On testing with a breathalyser, the police were surprised to see a reading that failed to register any alcohol and their perplexity increased when the man informed them he was a celebrated ballet dancer and had been going for a walk as a form of exercise and stamina building. The man was well-dressed and articulate, but had trouble sitting still while telling his story, and his squirming movements coupled with increasing agitation confirmed the police's impression that something 'fishy' was going on. When he spilled a cup of scalding hot coffee over his clothes and hands, the officer on duty surmised the man was 'on something' and he was brought to hospital for a medical check-up before being formally charged with creating a public nuisance.

On arrival in the Emergency Room, the man's agitation became pronounced and he tried to abscond, claiming the Central Intelligence Agency was behind a plot to have him silenced. This startling revelation led to a psychiatric consult and the police quietly withdrawing from the scene. To calm the agitation and reduce the risk of flight, a 2 mg intramuscular injection of haloperidol was given. This rapidly settled the restlessness and apart from some fidgity hand movements, the patient's appearance was unremarkable. His mental state, however, was anything but. He initially refused to talk to a psychiatrist, but once he realized that he would not be going home for the night and had been brought dinner and some hospital pyjamas, he began telling a tale composed of elaborate persecutory and grandiose delusions.

He claimed to have found a cure for AIDS and was being hounded by the CIA who wanted his secret. To avoid capture, he had been traveling between Canada and the United States, crossing the border whenever he felt the secret service of one of the countries was closing in on him. When questioned about his private life, stated he was single, had once been a professional dancer and choreographer, but had not worked in years, lived off the charity of friends, slept in their apartments or in hostels, and had no family, apart from an aged mother in a retirement home. Subsequent telephone calls to four friends and his mother confirmed all these facts to be true. Neither his mother nor friends were aware of his beliefs concerning the CIA and his professed cure for AIDS. However, they were all worried by his steady downward social drift, but could offer no explanation for it.

Two days following admission, his abnormal movements became more apparent. These were subtle, but writhing in nature. Gait was once again unsteady. The patient denied awareness of these problems, but agreed to a full neurological examination, which added little to these initial observations. A detailed family history revealed that the patient's father had died from natural causes in his seventies. The patient had no siblings. There was no history of similar movements in a relative and no family history of mental illness. A brain CT scan was normal, but functional neuroimaging demonstrated marked hypoperfusion in the basal ganglia bilaterally (Figure 8.4). A subsequent brain MRI scan suggested some mild ventricular enlargement confined to the lateral horns of the anterior ventricles and pointed towards possible subtle atrophy of the head of the caudate nucleus. Despite the absence of a family history of Huntington's disease, the possibility of this diagnosis and the need for

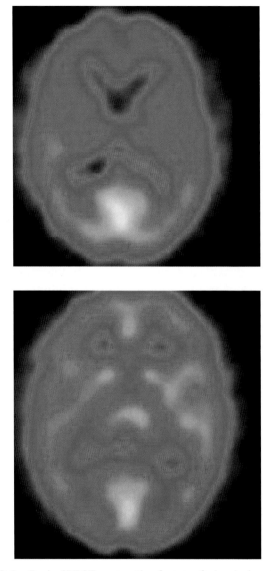

Figure 8.4 *Brain SPECT contrasting hypoperfusion in basal ganglia and frontal areas in a patient with Huntington's disease (top) with normal blood flow in a healthy control subject (bottom).*

genetic testing were discussed with the patient. He readily agreed to the blood test with an insouiance that conveyed the impression that we were all wasting out time – the problem lay with the CIA, not Mr Huntington, as far as he was concerned.

Genetic testing revealed the diagnosis of Huntingtons's disease, the case probably representing a spontaneous mutation in the sequence of cytosine–adenine–guanine repeats. In normal cases, the length of this sequence ends between 11 and 34 repeats, but in our patient the number was 37. Other possible explanations for the development of the disease included the family's suppressing knowledge of relatives with the condition or uncertainty over paternity. The former was considered unlikely, given the small number of known relatives, while exploring the latter was not an option.

The case therefore presented a number of interesting points, including the probable spontaneous mutation of the trinucleotide sequence, the florid early psychotic manifestation of Huntington's disease, the marked SPECT changes that contrasted with a normal CT brain scan and the subtlest MRI brain changes. The patient refused neuropsychological examination.

Case report 3

A man of Middle Eastern origin, in his mid-thirties, first presented at a neurological service complaining of poor vision and difficulty walking. It soon became apparent, however, that he had other difficulties relating to his mental state. He claimed that his problems began after he fell out of an airplane and floated 7000 metres to earth. Other outlandish statements included the assertion that he had breast fed his twin daughters, that his father was 136 years old and went for a run every morning in the desert accompanied by seven Arabian steeds. Should one of the horses tire, his father would pick up the animal and carry it home. The patient stated repeatedly that he was born in a Polish *shtetl* and spoke Yiddish, despite immigration papers that gave his country of origin as Iraq. What was noteworthy about these statements was that they remained consistent, the content never varying, although each time one had a conversation with him new and fantastic statements were forthcoming. The patient was oblivious to the incredulity his stories induced in his listeners.

Obtaining a factual history was difficult, for most answers were embellished with fantastical details. Thus, even ascertaining his exact age was difficult, given his claim that he had multiple birth certificates, all of which recorded different ages. What was known, however, through the Welfare offices and a copy of his divorce settlement, was that he was born in 1951, had lived alone since his divorce 5 years back and had not worked during this period. A transcript of the divorce proceedings revealed no evidence of confabulation.

The patient presented in a wheelchair, stating he could not stand or walk because of lower limb weakness. He was wearing a large pair of dark sunglasses and carried a white cane, claiming he was blind. On neurological examination, bilateral optic atrophy and extensor planter responses were noted. A mental state examination revealed a slightly obese, disheveled middle-aged male, whose behavior varied between apathy and social inappropriateness. When left alone in his room, he displayed little activity, sitting quietly in his wheelchair for hours. However, when in a busy day-area he became lively and made grossly inappropriate sexual approaches to female nursing staff and patients.

Prompted by his abnormal neurological examination an MRI scan of the brain and spinal cord was performed. The spine was normal, but brain images revealed a number of high signal confluent periventricular lesions (Figure 8.5) plus some discrete lesions. The lesion volume and distribution were quantified. Of a total brain lesion volume of 25.63 cm^3, 53% was distributed in the frontal lobes. Of greater significance, given the behavioral observations, was the presence of cerebral atrophy that was particularly prominent in bilateral frontal areas (Figure 8.6). Thus, not only were the frontal lobes more atrophied than other areas, but a little over half the lesion burden was frontally distributed. A mid-sagittal slice showed multiple lesions in an atrophied corpus callosum, giving the structure a 'punched-out' appearance (Figure 8.7). Consonant with the MRI result, the brain SPECT revealed marked frontal hypoperfusion (Figure 8.8).

Cerebrospinal fluid (CSF) analysis revealed normal protein and glucose levels and a single white blood cell, but was 2+ for oligoclonal banding while bilateral visual, right brain stem and somatosensory (right arm and leg) evoked potential readings were abnormal. Testing for syphilis (VDRL) was normal, as was an arylsulfatase level, ruling out the possibility of metachromatic leukodystrophy as part of the differential clinical diagnosis. All other blood tests were normal, including a full blood count and differential, electrolytes and urea and indices of a possible vasculitis, i.e. sedimentation rate, rheumatoid factor, antinuclear factor and complement levels. Cerebral angiography was not considered an option, given the above results.

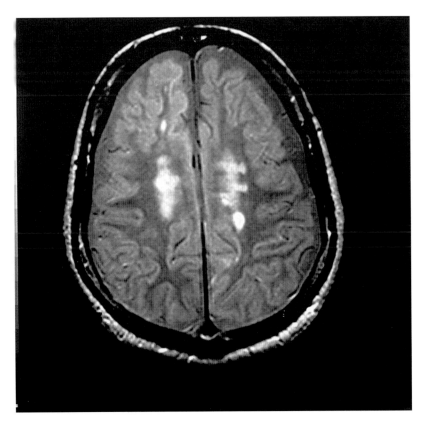

Figure 8.5 *Brain MRI in a man with multiple sclerosis and fantastic confabulations: confluent high signal periventricular abnormalities.*

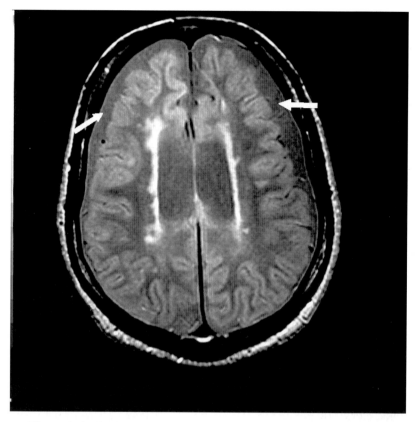

Figure 8.6 *Brain MRI in a man with multiple sclerosis and fantastic confabulations showing, in addition to periventricular lesions, significant bilateral frontal atrophy.*

Neuropsychological testing

The patient's score on the MMSE was 24/27 (the parts requiring vision were not administered). Other than hospital name, which was given as another local hospital, he was fully oriented. His recounting of recent political events was quite lucid, touching on local and national politics. He was able to name all but one of the major candidates in the national election. He used French, Italian, Portuguese and Arabic words and maintained a brief conversation in Portuguese with one of the examiners. Owing to his poor visual acuity, some tests were limited or administered in a non-standard fashion.

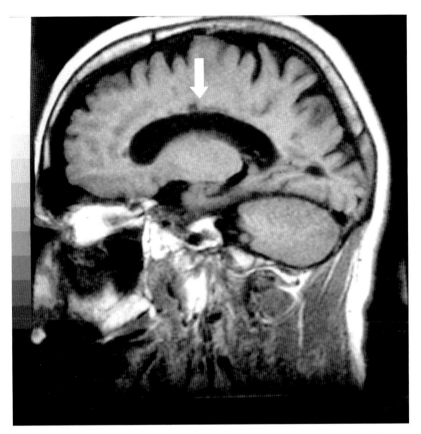

Figure 8.7 *Sagittal brain magnetic resonance image in a man with multiple sclerosis and fantastic confabulations, showing lesions in the corpus callosum.*

His prorated verbal IQ on the Wechsler Adult Intelligence Scale Revised (WAIS-R) (Wechsler, 1981), assuming an age range of 45–54 years, was 92, placing him at the low end of the average range. His spontaneous speech was fluent and well articulated with some mild word-finding problems. His simple comprehension was intact. Repetition was impaired only on long sentences demanding attention. His performance on the 'FAS' test was moderately impaired (Benton, 1968). On memory testing, acquisition of verbal material on the California Verbal Learning Test (CVLT) (Delis et al, 1987) and the Wechsler Memory Scale Revised

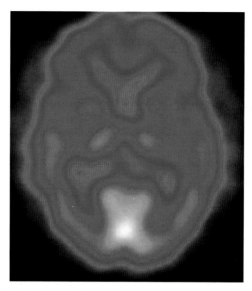

Figure 8.8   *Brain SPECT in a man with multiple sclerosis and fantastic confabulations, showing marked frontal hypoperfusion bilaterally.*

(WMS-R) (Wechsler, 1987) ranged from borderline to impaired and was lower than expected, given his verbal abilities. He accurately recalled and recognized information across the two testing sessions. As most tests traditionally used to assess executive function involve visual stimuli, executive assessment in this patient was limited to verbal abstract conceptual problems and analysis of his approach to the other neuro-psychological tests, which were generally concrete and stimulus-bound. For example, the proverb 'Rome was not built in a day' was interpreted as 'Rome was a huge city. It wasn't built in a day'.

In summary, testing was limited by his visual difficulties, but certain consistent findings emerged nevertheless. His most significant cognitive deficit was an inability to maintain focused, regulated information pro-cessing. Lack of regulation could also be observed in his mood and response to the testing demands. Although memory deficits were present, there was no loss of information or impaired everyday memory, and the nature and extent of the deficits were not those of a severe amnesic syndrome. In this regard, it was significant that delayed recall on the Wechsler Memory Scale was not impaired.

Bringing all the clinical, imaging, biochemical and neuropsychological strands together, there was little doubt that our patient had multiple sclerosis. Despite the exaggerated and inconsistent nature of his disability, the neurological examination revealed signs of two separate lesions in the central nervous system, namely optic atrophy and an extensor planter response. In addition to these clinical signs, paraclinical evidence (abnormal MRI and evoked potential results) plus laboratory data (2+ CSF oligoclonal banding) were in themselves strongly suggestive of demyelination.

The temporal sequence of how the symptoms had developed was unclear, but there was reason to believe from a copy of his divorce settlement 5 years earlier that confabulation was not present at that time. According to his ex-wife's testimony, however, disinhibited behavior was present and was instrumental in her desire for a separation. No mention was made of any physical difficulties. Thus, behavioral change may well have been the first sign of his multiple sclerosis. What makes the case unusual was not just the nature of the man's confabulations, but the fact that his 'pseudologica fantastica' occurred in the context of multiple sclerosis. This presentation of multiple sclerosis had not been previously reported and it was the results of the brain imaging that gave insights into the reasons for his atypical mentation.

There is a large literature describing confabulation in the context of severe memory difficulties, in particular the amnesic state most often noted in patients with Korsakoff psychosis (Shapiro et al, 1981; Victor et al, 1988). The confabulation is explained on the basis of the patients' attempts to compensate for their memory difficulties by filling in the gaps of their recall with made-up, but incorrect, information (Barbizet, 1963). However, not all confabulators are amnesic. Stuss et al (1978) have delineated two forms of confabulation in patients with neurological disorders: the amnesic patient whose responses are, for the most part, unremarkable; and the non-amnesic patient, whose less severe memory difficulties are accompanied by confabulations that are extravagantly fanciful. This second group displays evidence of marked frontal lobe dysfunction demonstrated by abnormalities on neuroimaging and neuropsychological testing. Patients of this sort are thought to have strategic retrieval deficits, particularly in the monitoring and verification of their own responses (Baddeley and Wilson, 1986; Moscovitch, 1989).

Should the amnesic picture be present, some reports suggest that additional frontal involvement, particularly in the ventromedial cortex, is a necessary prerequisite for associated confabulation (Moscovitch and Melo, 1997). A published case report using serial functional imaging supports this observation (Benson et al, 1996). A single amnesic subject underwent a SPECT brain scan while in a confabulatory state and thereafter had a repeat SPECT scan 4 months later, by which stage confabulation, but not the amnesic disorder, had stopped. Hypoperfusion of the orbital and medial frontal regions noted in the first scan was no longer present, although diencephalic hypoperfusion persisted. The cessation of confabulation and resolution of the frontal perfusion deficits were accompanied by similar improvements in performance on frontal lobe cognitive tests.

The data on our patient have many similarities to those described above. Memory deficits were apparent, but were not compatible with a pronounced amnesic syndrome. Neuropsychological paradigms probing frontal lobe function, such as the Wisconsin Card Sort Test, could not be given because of visual difficulties, but our patient's impaired verbal fluency and concrete responses to proverb interpretation, together with some perseverative responses, suggested frontal difficulties. The MRI data demonstrated subcortical white matter lesions with over 50% frontally distributed. Furthermore, significant cerebral atrophy was present, again mainly over the frontal convexities and in the region of the frontal interhemispheric fissure. Finally, frontal cerebral blood flow was markedly reduced.

It is not, however, clear why some, but not other patients with frontal lobe pathology confabulate. Berlyne (1972) has advanced a psychological explanation positing premorbid personality factors as potential modifiers of the process. While it would be shortsighted for any clinician to arrive at conclusions concerning a patient's mental state without recourse to psychosocial data, this explanation is inadequate. Rather, it probably requires a particular constellation of frontally mediated cognitive and behavioral features to coalesce before confabulation manifests.

References

Baddeley A, Wilson B (1986) Amnesia, autobiographical memory, and confabulation. In Rubin DC (ed) *Autobiographical Memory*. Cambridge: Cambridge University Press, 225–252.

Barbizet J (1963) Defect of memorizing of hippocampal-mamillary origin: a review. *J Neurol Neurosurg Psychiatry* **26**:127–135.

Bechara A, Damasio AR, Damasio H et al (1994) Insensitivity to future consequences following damage to human prefrontal cortex. *Cognition* **50**:7–15.

Benson DF, Djenderedjian A, Miller BL, Pachana NA, Chang L et al (1996) Neural basis of confabulation. *Neurology* **46**:1239–1243.

Benton AL (1968) Differential behavioral effects in frontal lobe disease. *Neuropsychologia* **6**:53–60.

Berlyne N (1972) Confabulation. *Br J Psychiatry* **120**:31–39.

Damasio A (1994) *Descarte's Error: Emotion, Reason and the Human Brain*. New York: Avon Science.

Delis DC, Kramer JH, Kaplan E, Ober BA (1987) *California Verbal Learning Test: Adult Version Manual*. San Antonio, TX: The Psychological Corporation.

Folstein MF, Folstein SE, McHugh PR (1975) 'Mini-Mental State': A practical method for grading the cognitive state of patients for the clinician. *J Psychiatr Res* **12**:189–198.

Gronwall DMA (1977) Paced Auditory Serial Addition Task: a measure of recovery from concussion. *Percept Motor Skills* **44**:367–373.

Harlow JM (1993) Classic Text No.4. Recovery from the passage of an ion bar through the head. *Hist Psychiatry* iv: 271–281.

Heaton RK (1981) *Wisconsin Card Sorting Test Manual*. Odessa, FL: Psychological Assessment Resources.

Moscovitch M (1989) Confabulation and the frontal systems: Strategic versus associative retrieval in neuropsychological theories of memory. In Roediger HL, Craik FIM (eds) *Varieties of Memory and Consciousness: Essays in Honour of Endel Tulving*. Hilldale, NJ: Lea, 1989:133–160.

Moscovitch M, Melo B (1997) Strategic retrieval and the frontal lobes: Evidence from confabulation and amnesia. *Neuropsychologia* **35**:1017–1034.

Shapiro BE, Alexander MP, Gardner H, Mercer B (1981) Mechanisms of confabulation. *Neurology* **31**:1070–1076.

Stuss DT, Alexander MP, Lieberman A, Levine H (1978) An extraordinary form of confabulation. *Neurology* **28**:1166–1172.

Victor M, Adams RD, Collins GH (1988) *The Wernicke-Korsakoff Syndrome*, 2nd Edn. Philadelphia: FA Davis.

Wechsler D (1981) *Wechsler Adult Intelligence Scale – Revised.* New York: Psychological Corporation.
Wechsler D (1987) *Wechsler Memory Scale – Revised.* San Antonio, TX: The Psychological Corporation.

Appendix 8.1

A most dramatic demonstration of the behavioral consequences of damage to the ventral prefrontal cortex is provided by the celebrated case of Phineas Gage, the New England railway worker who sustained a grievous traumatic brain injury. Gage's physician was John Martyn Harlow (1819–1907), who wrote two reports on his patient, the first within weeks of the injury and the second, a year later, describing the changes in behavior he noted. A summary of Dr Harlow's observations is informative.

'The accident occurred in Cavendish, VT on the line of the Rutland and Burtlington Railroad, at that time being built, on the 13th of September 1848, and was occasioned by the premature explosion of a blast, when this iron, known to blasters as a tamping iron, ... was shot through the face and head ... The iron is 3 feet 7 inches in length and weighs 13 and one fourth pounds ... The patient was thrown back by the explosion, and gave a few convulsive motions of the extremities, but spoke in a few minutes. His men (with whom he was a great favorite) took him in their arms and carried him to the road ... put him in an ox cart in which he rode, supported in a sitting posture, fully three quarters of a mile to his hotel. He got out of the car himself, with a little assistance from his men and an hour afterwards walked up a long flight of stairs ... he seemed perfectly conscious, but was becoming exhausted from the hemorrhage ... he bore his sufferings with firmness, and directed my attention to the hole in his cheek, saying, 'the iron entered there and passed through my head.'

In tending to the wound, Dr Harlow wrote, 'I passed the index finger of the right hand into the opening it's entire length, in the direction of the wound in the cheek, which received the left index finger in like manner, the introduction of the finger into the brain being scarcely felt.'

Remarkable as these observations are, it is Harlow's later behavioral observations that have assured Phineas Gage's place among the most celebrated of case histories. Writing of a visit Gage made to him in April 1849, he observed the following: 'General appearance good; stands quite erect, ... his gait is steady, his movements rapid and easily executed ... can adduct and depress the globe, but cannot move it in other directions; vision lost ... upon the top of the head and covered with hair, is a large unequal depression and elevation – a quadrangular fragment of bone, which was entirely detached from the frontal, and extending low upon the forehead, being still raised and quite prominent. His physical health is good and I am inclined to say that he has recovered ... His contractors, who regarded him as the most efficient and capable foreman in their employ previous to his injury, considered the change in his mind so marked that they could not give him his place again. The equilibrium or balance, so to speak, between his intellectual faculties and animal propensities, seems to have been destroyed. He is fitful, irreverent, indulging at times in the grossest profanity (which was not previously his custom), manifesting but little deference to his fellows, impatient of restraint or advice when it conflicts with his desires, at times pertinaciously obstinate, yet capricious and vacillating, devising many plans of future operation, which are no sooner arranged than they are abandoned in turn for others appearing more feasible. A child of his intellectual capacity and manifestations, he has the animal passions of a strong man. Previous to his injury, though untrained in the schools, he possessed a well balanced mind, and was looked upon by those who knew him as a shrewd, smart business man, very energetic and persistent in executing all his plans of operation. In this regard, his mind was radically changed, so decidedly that his friends and acquaintances said he was no longer Gage.'

chapter 9

Clinical vignettes

Case 1 'Clock drawing and recovery from delirium'

A 75-year-old widower was admitted to a chronic care hospital following a major stroke causing right-sided hemiplegia. In the post-stroke period he was noted to be emotionally labile and tearful and was started on amitriptyline with increasing doses up to 150 mg daily. Psychiatric consultation was requested because of persistent lability and mood symptomatology. On initial assessment, he showed evidence of marked disorientation to time and place. He was in a hospital in London, England and while sitting in front of the lift (elevator) he imagined that he was in a tube (subway) station.

Among the cognitive screening tests done was the clock drawing test (Figure 9.1). The initial clock shows evidence of marked visuospatial impairment and extremely poor planning. He also showed evidence of perseveration and concrete thinking when asked to denote the time at 3 o'clock. Inattention is evident by the omission of the number 9. A provisional diagnosis of toxic delirium secondary to tricyclic antidepressants was established and the medication was discontinued.

He was then reassessed 2 weeks later and showed a significant improvement in his mental state and level of alertness. He was now much better oriented and integrated in his clinical presentation. The clock drawing test was repeated 2 weeks later and a significant improve-

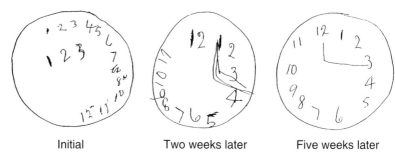

| Initial | Two weeks later | Five weeks later |

Figure 9.1 *Improvement following toxic delirium. (Reproduced from Shulman et al, 1986, with permission from John Wiley & Sons Ltd.)*

ment in his planning ability was evident, although he still showed residual impairment. While he was now able to denote time using hands, he showed evidence of perseveration as a result of the residual cognitive impairment. However, 5 weeks later, when he was very dramatically improved from a clinical perspective, his clock drawing test also reflected significant improvement. He was able to draw virtually a perfect clock with excellent visuospatial organization and was able to denote 3 o'clock accurately.

Summary

The visual representation of the improvement in his central nervous system function had a significant impact on the treating team, who were able to recognize very quickly that indeed the anticholinergic toxicity resulting from tricyclic treatment was the clear etiology of his impairment. Moreover, its discontinuation was responsible for his significant improvement. The clock drawing test proved to be sensitive to cognitive change and an efficient practical tool for use on a medical ward.

Case 2   'Cognitive screening vs detailed neuropsychiatric assessment in a complex case'

A 75-year-old retired professor was seen for psychiatric consultation because of persistent headaches as well as depressive and anxiety symptoms. She had a very complex history that included, hypothyroidism, mild hepatic dysfunction and a history of narcotic analgesic use for persistent headaches. Her mother suffered from late-onset headaches which eventually developed into a progressive dementia.

Brief cognitive screening (2000–2003)
The cognitive screening tests, clock drawing and Mini Mental State Examination (MMSE), demonstrated a pattern of fluctuations yet overall deterioration. Of interest is the fact that detailed neurosychological testing (see below) was not any more elucidating of the nature of her condition. A series of clock drawings from March 2000 to February 2003 showed evidence of deterioration (Figure 9.2). The first clock shows evidence of good visuospatial organization and an

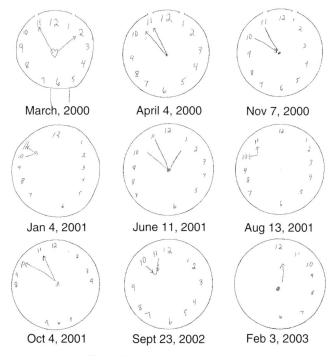

Figure 9.2   Consecutive clocks.

accurate denotation of time at 10 past 11. Within 1 month, however, her second clock test reveals a frontal pull to the 10 while there is still preservation of visuospatial ability. In May of the same year, there was more subtle impairment in the spacing of the numbers and an attempt to correct the 11:10 denotation. She still showed inaccuracy in denoting time by pointing the minute hand to the 1 instead of the 2 and the hour hand pointing just after the 10. Some 6 months later, in November 2000, her clock again reverted to the frontal pull with arrows pointing in the wrong direction and some mild spacing difficulties now evident. In January 2001 her clock drawing was more fragmented in terms of spacing as well as in her denotation of time. Six months later, in June 2001, her spacing continued to be some-what fragmented and she showed ambivalence in her denotation of time but still with a frontal pull. By August 2001 the same pattern persisted until October 2001, when the spacing fragmentation was more severely impaired and the pull to 10 past 11 continued.

A significant deterioration in her MMSE score occurred in August 2001 down to 23/30, whereas in the year previously (2000) she had scored 28/30 on the MMSE. By August 2002 the MMSE score was 20/30 and she was now more clearly dementing. Further assessment in December 2002 revealed an MMSE score of 16/30.

Detailed neurological, psychiatric and neuropsychological testing
May 2000
Detailed neuropsychological testing reflected the inconclusive nature of her condition. The assessors postulated three potential causes of her cognitive dysfunction: depression, hypothyroidism and early dementia.

Her full-scale IQ was in the average range and the Dementia Rating Scale was within normal limits. She scored low average on some of the executive tasks and showed impairment on psychomotor tasks including trail making A and B. Her Boston naming task was impaired as well as short-term verbal and non-verbal learning and recall. Visual constructive tasks were considered to be within normal limits.

August 2000

A detailed **cognitive neurology** assessment noted problems with attention, especially backward digit span, short-term verbal memory and visual memory. However, her remote memory remained reasonably intact and language tasks were considered to be intact. She was unable to draw a cube and showed frontal pull on the clock drawing test. There was evidence of concrete interpretation on tasks of abstraction and she had difficulty with the Luria sequences. Word-list generation for phonemically cued words was 15 as well as for semantically cued words. The neurology assessment was equivocal: '*All of the above are compatible with probable Alzheimer's disease, but mood, anxiety and chronic pain are contributing factors*'. A trial of the cholinesterase inhibitor donepezil was instituted at that time.

February 2001

A **headache (neurology) specialist** was consulted but a review of the magnetic resonance imaging and single photo emission computed tomography scan did not reveal any clear neurological disorder or lesion. The conclusion was that '*her headaches must be somatic manifestations of depression and I would suggest a trial of MAO inhibitors since these drugs may be very effective in this situation.*'

August 2001

A **stroke neurologist** assessed the patient after she was brought to the emergency room with an acute confusional state. This neurologist had the following opinion: '*On examination, I found her neurologically normal except on psychological testing. I found her answers to many of the questions of naming and clock drawing to be inappropriate and* **not compatible with an organic confusional state**. *For instance, she drew the clock rapidly and accurately but then put the hands at 11 and 5 when asked to draw 5 past 11. She became tearful at one point during the questioning. Her orientation, however, was excellent and her long-term memory was excellent though her short-term memory appears to show difficulties in concentration. I believe all the patient's problems can be explained on the basis of depression.*'

November 2001

She was seen by a second **behavioral neurologist** because of the possibility of Lewy body dementia subsequent to a number of episodes in which she complained of visual hallucinations. The behavioral neurologist formed a final opinion of '*differential diagnosis as Lewy body disease versus depression.*' This neurologist suggested a switch to a different cholinesterase inhibitor in the form of galantamine, aggressive treatment of depression as well as detailed neuropsychological testing.

Mental Status Examination during the **behavioral neurology assessment** was as follows: '*She was appropriate and co-operative. On tests of memory she did well. She was oriented to year, month, day and date. She knew who the Prime Minister of Canada was but not who the Premier of Ontario was. She was able to recall 3/3 items at 5 minutes and again at 10 minutes. She had difficulty on tests of attention and concentration. She was unable to do serial 7's subtraction. She was markedly impaired on reciting months of the year in reverse order. She was able to do serial 3's subtraction and spell the word "world" backwards. On tests of language, her spontaneous speech, auditory comprehension, repetition and naming were intact.*

Clock drawing was poor to command. On her free-drawn clock she drew the numbers in reverse order. For 10 after 11:00 she put a hand at the 10 and at the 11. On the examiner's clock she also set the hands at 10 to 11:00. In contrast, her clock drawing to copy was quite good and was significantly better than her clock drawing to command.

On tests of visuo-spatial function her drawing of a house was good except that it lacked 3-dimensional perspective. Drawing of a cube also lacked 3-dimensional perspective. Drawing to copy of a house and the intersecting pentagons was adequate. On tests of abstraction she had difficulty on the harder similarities items and on 1 out of 2 proverbs. She perseverated on drawing alternating square and triangular figures but not on multiple loops. Word list generation for words beginning with the letter "F" was 14 and for animal names it was 9 (this was lower than August, 2001). There was no ideomotor apraxia for limb, buccofacial and whole body commands.

Opinion

Mrs. X is a 70 year old woman with an approximately 3-year history of depression and headache. She also has difficulty with cognition on history and has had 3 episodes of hallucinations. Her Mental Status Examination is remarkable for marked deficits in attention. She also showed perseveration. Her clock drawing is also poor. In addition she had difficulty with verbal fluency, especially for animal names. Manipulation of information as tested by proverb and similarities was also mildly impaired.

The differential diagnosis lies between Lewy body disease vs Depression. With respect to Lewy body disease, features that go along with this disorder on mental status testing are her prominent attentional deficits in the setting of good performance on memory tasks. Her verbal fluency, especially for animals, is also typical for Lewy body disease. In contrast, her clock drawing to copy improved and this is said to be atypical for this disorder. Nevertheless, Lewy body disease still needs to be considered.'

Because of persistent and intractable depressive symptoms and co-morbid headaches, she was seen by a **psychiatrist with expertise in transcranial magnetic stimulation** (TMS).

With respect to diagnosis, there is little doubt that she suffers from at least two conditions, one of them and the more compelling of the two, being of neurological origin. Diagnoses of Lewy Body Disease and Alzheimer's Disease have been offered. She would, at this time, meet criteria for Major Depressive Disorder. It is possible that her dementia is actually a pseudo-dementia, but this is rather unlikely given the insidious deteriorating course and the family history of dementia. The differential diagnosis would include Mood Disorder secondary to other medical pathology such as thyroid dysfunction, medication toxicity, metabolic derangement of some type (her sodium levels have been low during several determinations, though I understand these are now normal), all of these being rather unlikely in the face of the extensive negative investigations.'

A subsequent course of TMS resulted in transient improvement only.

January 2002

Follow-up in the **cognitive neurology clinic** revealed that *'the underlying basis of her memory complaints remains unclear. I think that Lewy Body Disease remains in the differential or it may be mild Alzheimer's disease. However, the picture is predominated by her depression and made worse by her headaches.'*

'Mrs. X was referred for assessment of her memory and cognitive functioning. Currently she is operating in the average range of intellectual functioning, with both her verbal and visual spatial reasoning skills well within average limits. On neuropsychological tests she exhibited a generalized decline of function across several cognitive domains. Relative weaknesses lie in her semantic memory, verbal learning, visual naming to confrontation, immediate and delayed visual recall and recognition, visual scanning speed and attention shifting which are in the borderline to impaired range. Visual construction, delayed verbal recall and recognition, and verbal fluency are low average to borderline, while attention/concentration and arithmetic skills are within the borderline range. Relative strengths include sustained auditory attention, practical problem solving/conceptual programming/manual praxis are observed. Mrs. X denied any depressive symptoms in a self-reported inventory of depression during testing.

Mrs. X's pattern of neuropsychological deficits is suggestive of generalized cognitive decline. A neurodegenerative process such as Alzheimer's disease cannot be ruled out although her pattern of deficits is more widespread than would be expected in this case. Given the absence of parkinsonian signs and the fact that her episodes of hallucination were apparently isolated incidents that have not recurred after discontinuation of certain medications, Lewy-body disease appears unlikely. Consideration should be given to a generalized systemic disorder as a cause of her cognitive problems. Although she has a history of depression and persistent headaches, these factors are not likely contributing to the overall neuropsychological picture to a significant degree.

May 2002

A second detailed **neuropsychological assessment** was conducted with the following test results:

Domain (Test name(s))	Results
Intellectual functioning (WAIS)	Full Scale IQ: average Vocabulary: average Visual spatial/matrix reasoning – average
Attention/Concentration (KBNA)	Mental sequences and spatial location: borderline
Verbal Learning (KBNA acquisition trials)	Impaired (learned 3/12 words by 4th learning trial)
Delayed Verbal Recall (KBNA)	Low average to borderline
Delayed Verbal Recognition (KBNA)	Low average
Immediate and Delayed Visual Recall (KBNA)	Borderline to impaired
Delayed Visual Recognition (KBNA)	Impaired
Visual Constructional Ability (KBNA Complex Figure; Clocks)	Low average
Visual scanning/attention speed (KBNA)	Impaired
Sustained auditory attention (KBNA)	Within normal limits
Visual Naming to Confrontation (KBNA)	Impaired
Word List Generation – Phonemic (KBNA)	Low average
Word List Generation – Semantic (KBNA animal and first names)	Low average to borderline
Arithmetic Skills (KBNA Arithmetic)	Borderline
Motor Programming and Manual Praxis (KBNA Praxis)	Within normal limits
Practical Reasoning (KBNA)	Within normal limits
Conceptual shifting (KBNA)	Within normal limits
Depression (BDI)	Within normal limits, denied any depressive symptoms
Visual tracking (Trails A and B speed/attention shifting	Impaired
Primary and working memory (WAIS-III Digits Span)	Average

Summary

This is an example of a complex case with multi-faceted aspects that remained unclear for a number of years. This case illustrates the difficulties of establishing a clear diagnosis with slowly progressive cognitive changes in the context of complex medical and psychiatric symptoms and multiple pharmacological treatments. The marked fluctuations in her clinical course are suggestive of a Lewy body dementia including episodes of hallucinations associated with certain psychotropic agents. However, her clinical condition remained unclear despite frequent follow-up by behavioral neurology, detailed neuropsychological testing and close medical follow-up. Aggressive antidepressant, cognitive and analgesic therapy was ineffective. During this past year her dementia became more obvious and her associated somatic symptoms and depression improved.

Brief cognitive testing (MMSE, clock drawing test and word fluency) was sufficient to highlight concerns about her cognitive functioning as well as documenting the fluctuations and deterioration in her clinical course. Detailed, neuropsychological testing in this situation did not add significantly to the understanding of the nature and etiology of this complex disorder.

Case 3 'Somatization and depressive symptoms as prodromal features of dementia'

An 81-year-old woman was seen in psychiatric consultation in July 1998 with symptoms of increasing somatization. There was no prior psychiatric history nor was there any family history of mental disorder. Her self-care was not as good as it had been and she had shown some loss of interest in her grandchildren, who previously had been a very important focus for her life. She was a very high functioning woman with outstanding intellect premorbidly.

The following findings were recorded at her initial cognitive assessment: '*Premorbidly this woman was of high native intelligence, but scored 27/30 on the Mini-Mental State Examination with impairment of recall*

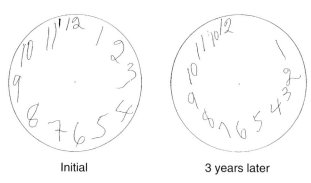

Initial   3 years later

Figure 9.3   *Deterioration in clock drawing.*

and concentration. She was also hesitant on a number of tasks. Clock drawing showed good visual–spatial organization and planning, but she was unable to correctly denote 11:10, pointing to a line just after 11:00 [Figure 9.3]. She was able to use hands to denote 3:00 accurately. Throughout the interview, there was evidence of some word finding difficulty. On formal testing, she showed impairment of abstraction as tested by similarities. She was only able to generate 6 words beginning with the letter "F" in 1 minute, and only 7 animals with some perseveration. She showed good right/left orientation, but had sensory extinction on bilateral stimulation on the face/hand test. She also struggled with simple calculation instructions. She insisted that her age was 80 even though she has just turned 81.

In summary, this 81-year-old woman presents with a one and a half to two year history of change in mental state, characterized by somatization and a decrease in her overall level of functioning with increasingly constricted lifestyle. On formal testing, the main finding is evidence of high level cognitive dysfunction. It is my opinion that the history and clinical presentation are consistent with a primary cognitive deficit, most likely a dementia of the Alzheimer type. At this point, appropriate neuroimaging needs to be undertaken and I am recommending that we do neuropsychological screening to further document the extent of her cognitive dysfunction and establish a baseline for follow-up. I also need to be reassured that she has had a good general medical screen, including a thyroid screen to ensure there is not a medical or systemic basis for her central nervous system disturbance.'

As a result of this initial consultation, a request was made for neuropsychological consultation. An interesting note was received the following month from the **neuropsychologist**. It highlights the problems in assessing someone of very high premorbid IQ. *'Mrs. X denied having any unusual memory or other cognitive problems and this was confirmed by Mr. X. Mr. X denied that his wife repeatedly asks questions, forgets information quickly, is disoriented to time, gets lost in familiar or unfamiliar surroundings or has significant word-finding problems. Mrs. X denied having a history of head injury, stroke, cardiac illness, hypertension, thyroid deficiency, diabetes or cancer. She is currently taking Zoloft and Ativan for "nervousness", although she reported that you have recommended that she gradually discontinue the Ativan. I discussed the reason and purpose of a neuropsychological assessment with the X's and they did not see any reason to proceed with the assessment given that Mrs. X is not experiencing any significant cognitive problems.'*

She was reassessed some 3 years later in July 2001. At that time, she had been followed by a neurologist for a now well-established dementia and was started on Donepezil, a cholinesterase inhibitor. Her MMSE was 21/30, whereas 3 years ago it was 28/30. Clock drawing also showed deterioration in that her initial clock demonstrated excellent visuospatial organization but an inability to denote 10 past 11 (Figure 9.3), whereas in July 2001 her clock drawing test revealed evidence of poor spacing and concrete response to the denotation of 11:10.

Summary

One should always be vigilant in assessing individuals who have high premorbid IQ and not make the mistake of the neuropsychologist in simply dismissing the concerns based on a lack of subjective impairment. The simple cognitive screening tests at initial assessment did raise concerns about a possible dementia at a time when functioning was still at a high level and the focus was on her somatization.

Case 4 'Manic delirium and recovery associated with chronic cardiac disease'

A retired dentist was referred for assessment following an episode of confusion and manic disinhibition during a recent hospitalization. He had a history of chronic coronary artery disease including heart failure, atrial fibrillation, cardiomyopathy and a history of two coronary artery bypass operations, two angioplasties and evidence of renal failure secondary to renal artery stenosis. There was a strong family history of vascular disease in the family.

Associated with the delirium was a clear manic syndrome followed by a mixed affective state with depressive features but evidence during the hospitalization of disinhibition, hyperloquaciousness, visual hallucinations, perseveration, poor judgement and emotional lability. He was treated with mood stabilizers with slow resolution.

At an initial psychiatric assessment following his hospitalization, the following cognitive examination was recorded: '*He scored 28/30 on the Mini-Mental State Examination. He recalled only two of three objects and thought we were on the second floor of the hospital when we were on the ground floor. Clock drawing test revealed only subtle impairment in his use of spacing [Figure 9.4]. Word fluency revealed that he was able to generate only ten words with the phonemic prime of "F" and 16 words with the semantic prime of four-legged animals. The remainder of the cognitive examination was within normal limits although typically he had very little recollection of the recent hospitalization consistent with his delirium.*'

Clinical course

Over the next few months, he continued to be treated on slowly tapering mood stabilizing medication. His clinical state gradually resolved after some fluctuations in his hypomanic and depressive symptomatology. Six months later, he was essentially back to his premorbid level. Repeat cognitive testing using screening instruments documented the clinically significant but subtle improvement on testing. The MMSE now improved to 30/30. Word fluency showed an improvement to 14 words

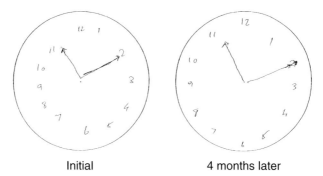

Initial   4 months later

Figure 9.4   *Subtle improvement in clock drawing.*

on phonemic prime of 'F' compared to 10 words at initial assessment. Word generation in response to the semantic prime of 'four-legged animals' increased to 18 from 16 and the clock drawing test showed an improvement in his use of spacing compared to the initial assessment (Figure 9.4). This was unlikely to be a practice effect as the testing was done 6 months after the initial assessment.

Summary

This case illustrates the sensitivity of cognitive screening instruments to cognitive change in an individual with very high premorbid IQ recovering from a manic delirium associated with cerebrovascular disease and significant cardiac disease. Despite the clear history of delirium, his cognitive assessment showed only subtle deficits, probably because of his very high premorbid level of intelligence and education. Nonetheless, the cognitive screening instruments proved to be cost-effective and acceptable methods of documenting cognition over time.

References

Shulman KI, Shedletsky R, Silver IL (1986). The challenge of time: Clock-drawing and cognitive function in the elderly. *Int J Geriatr Psychiatry* **1**:135–140.

Index